D0168449

Paul O'Brien, MD

THE LAP-BAND™
SOLUTION

A Partnership in Weight Loss
An Information Book

**The Centre for Bariatric
Surgery, Melbourne, Australia
and The American Institute of
Gastric Banding, Dallas USA**

MUP | C

Melbourne University Publishing

MUP CUSTOM
An imprint of Melbourne University Publishing Ltd
187 Grattan Street, Carlton, Victoria 3053, Australia
mup-custom@unimelb.edu.au
www.mup.com.au

First published 2007
Text © Paul O'Brien 2007
Images © individual copyright holders 2007
Design and typography © Melbourne University Publishing Ltd
2007

Designed by Catherine Nolan Biondic
Typeset in Malaysia by Syarikat Seng Teik
Printed in Australia by Griffin Press

National Library of Australia Cataloguing-in-Publication entry

O'Brien, Paul (Paul Edmond), 1943– .
    The lap band solution: a partnership for weight loss.

    1st ed.
    Bibliography.
    Includes index.
    ISBN 9780522854121.

    1. Obesity—Surgery. 2. Stomach—Surgery.
    3. Weight loss—Surgery. I. Title.

617.43

FOREWORD

When Dr O'Brien first told me of his plans to write a book about the LAP-BAND™, I was delighted. Not only is he a gifted surgeon and the world's foremost authority, but a compassionate, kind man who genuinely cares about the health and welfare of people struggling with their weight.

You, the reader, are to be commended for taking the initiative to learn more about the remarkable LAP-BAND™ system and how this simple device can change your life. Whether you are considering having the procedure or already have the band and want to optimize your success, this book provides the information you need in a clear and concise manner.

Those of us involved with LAP-BAND™ surgery in the United States have always looked to our colleagues in Australia because of their much longer experience with the procedure, as well as the outstanding weight loss achieved by their patients. As I spoke with Dr O'Brien and observed his interaction with his patients, the importance of a structured aftercare program became clearly apparent. I encourage you to look at the LAP-BAND™ as a tool—remarkable, yes, but still a tool.

The key to success with any tool is understanding how it works and the things you as a patient can do to make it work better for *you*.

This book will serve as an owner's manual and road map as you begin your journey to a happier, healthier lifestyle. Best of luck and enjoy the trip.

Peter R. Gottlieb
Founder and Director
The American Institute of Gastric Banding

ABOUT THE AUTHOR

 Paul O'Brien is a world leader in the LAP-BAND™ procedure. He was one of its originators, having been involved in its design and testing in the early 1990s, and he placed the first LAP-BAND™ in Australia in 1994. He is the Head of the Centre for Bariatric Surgery (CBS), a major clinical center for the assessment and treatment of obesity in Melbourne, Australia (Web site: <www.lapbandaustralia.com.au>). The center has six surgeons, seven physicians and nine other health professionals committed to providing a safe and effective weight loss program and, by the end of 2006, had treated more than 3,500 patients with the LAP-BAND™.

He is also Emeritus Professor of Surgery at Monash University and the Director of the Centre for Obesity Research and Education (CORE), a major research center within Monash University in Melbourne (Web site: <www.core.monash.org>). His principal areas of clinical and research interest are in the morbidity of obesity and the health benefits of weight loss. He has published more than 200 research papers in the medical literature and has been active in conducting numerous postgraduate courses and workshops on obesity and its treatments in Australia, the United States, countries of the Asia–Pacific region, South America and Canada.

He is Past President of the Obesity Surgery Society of Australia and New Zealand (1997–2004). He was President of the 11th World Congress of the International Federation for the Surgery of Obesity (IFSO), held in Sydney, Australia in August/September, 2006. He is the Co-Editor-in-Chief of the journal *Obesity Surgery*, the leading journal for the science of weight loss surgery, and one of the leading surgical journals in the world.

He has recently taken the position of National Medical Director for the American Institute for Gastric Banding (AIGB), in Dallas, Texas (Web site: <www.aigb.com>). This is the most active and experienced clinical group in the United States for providing the LAP-BAND™ in a day surgery setting, and more than 7,500 patients have been treated. In association with Dr O'Brien, it is rapidly expanding to provide a comprehensive treatment and follow-up service across the United States.

He lives in Melbourne with his wife, Eve, and near their four grown-up children Tim, Charlotte, Richard and Anna.

CONTENTS

ACKNOWLEDGMENTS

I would like to thank our patients who, by telling us how they feel, have taught us so much. They have been so keen, so supportive and so tolerant. Hopefully we have been able to contribute to their health and happiness as a result.

The staff of the Centre for Bariatric Surgery have been invaluable in working together to find the optimal program of care. In particular, Chris Halkett, one of our Nurse Coordinators, has worked closely with me since we began the program in 1994, and knows our patients better than I, providing advice and reassurance for them day and night. Kathy Noble coordinated the program in the early days and contributed greatly.

I am very grateful to the other surgeons of the group—Drs Wendy Brown, Stewart Skinnner, Stephen Blamey, Gary Crosthwaite and Andrew Smith—for their skillful support and commitment to excellent patient care.

Our medical aftercare team began when Dr Audrey Kotzander joined me in 1997 and now also includes Drs John Dixon, Anna Korin, Peter Baquie, Paul Macartney and Kathryn De Garis as Primary Care

Practitioners, and Linda Schachter and Friederike Veit as Specialist Physicians. Much of our understanding of the aftercare needs has been developed from discussions with these colleagues.

Cheryl Laurie, Robyn Bowyer, Julie Playfair and Eve O'Brien provide the nursing support and collect great insights through their close contact with our patients. Susan Colles, Meagan Walker, Colleen Ash and Melissa McGrice provide the invaluable perspective of the dietician. Margaret Anderson has maintained the database that is central to the aftercare of our patients, tracking their progress and measuring their outcomes.

Through the Centre for Obesity Research and Education we have observed, measured, analyzed and studied many aspects of the problems of obesity, and the benefits of weight loss and the LAP-BAND™ process. John Dixon has been central to these studies and we have been assisted by our research nurses, Cheryl Laurie and Julie Playfair, and by Veronica Alvarez-Vliegenthart, Maureen Dixon, Andrew Dixon, Timothy Chaston and Tracey McPhail.

A key feature of successful LAP-BAND™ practice is the coordinated involvement of a multidisciplinary team, and the successful patient outcomes of the Centre for Bariatric Surgery are a credit to them all.

INTRODUCTION

This book has been written for two groups of people. Firstly, it is written for those people who have a problem with their weight and are wanting to be informed about the LAP-BAND™ as one of the major options for treatment.

Secondly, it is written for the people who have made the decision to proceed with the LAP-BAND™ procedure and need to know what will happen at the time of surgery, what are the guidelines for eating, exercise and lifestyle, and how they can contribute to achieving an optimal outcome.

It is not necessary to read the book "from cover to cover." You can if you wish but that is not our expectation. We would like you to read different parts at different stages of your progress from the initial exploration of the possibility of having the LAP-BAND™ through to your days, months and years after placement of the band and the learning of a new way of life. Read the key parts for each stage as you progress. Over the years after the surgery, read the chapters on eating and exercise again and again to be sure you are fully familiar with them and are following the advice.

The first two chapters provide background information about the problem of obesity and the benefits of weight loss. Many people who come to see us are already well informed on these matters. It may be that much of the material in these two chapters is already known to you. Please look through it. See if there is new information. See if the information presented gives you a better understanding of your problem and your options. The decision to have the LAP-BAND™ is one of the most important healthcare decisions that you will make and it is best to make that decision on the basis of good information and understanding. These two chapters are there to provide that information.

Chapter 3 reviews the options available to you if you have the disease of obesity. It is an overview rather than a detailed review of treatments. We give enough information about each of the treatment options to clarify why we are or are not expecting that treatment to be your best option. For someone who is starting the process of exploring the treatments available for weight reduction, this chapter should be helpful. It does not attempt to provide a comprehensive review of all the other options. That is for others to provide. Rather, it focuses on why we see the LAP-BAND™ as the best option for the primary treatment of the disease of obesity.

Chapter 4 provides detailed information about the LAP-BAND™. It covers the key advantages that the

LAP-BAND™ provides over other options. It reviews the good outcomes and the possible bad outcomes. It ends with a synthesis of the attributes of all the other possible treatments for obesity in comparison with the LAP-BAND™.

Chapter 5 and subsequent chapters are for you once you have decided to go ahead with the LAP-BAND™. This chapter tells you what you need to know about your time in hospital and the first 4 weeks after operation. By that time, you will be over the operation, the band will be settling into position and you are ready to start the phase of serious weight reduction.

Chapters 6 and 7 provide details of the rules and guidelines relating to eating, drinking, exercise and activity that are recommended to be followed with the LAP-BAND™. These are the two most important chapters in the book. We want you to read them carefully and read them several times if you are planning to go ahead with the procedure.

Chapter 8 informs you about the adjustment sequence. It explains how we determine when to add fluid, how much to add, and what happens to your appetite in association with adjustments. The adjustability of the band is its most important attribute. We use it with enthusiasm but with careful judgment.

Chapter 9 tells you what should happen with your weight as we adjust the band and as you follow the eating and exercise guidelines. It tells you how much weight you are most likely to lose, how quickly you should lose it, what we do if you are losing weight more slowly than we expected and what you can do to optimize the effectiveness of the band.

Chapter 10 summarizes the guidelines into eight golden rules. We encourage you to treat these rules as critical to achieving the best possible result from the LAP-BAND™.

Chapter 11 addresses the many questions that are put to us. It repeats many parts of the earlier chapters but does represent what people worry about. It is worth reading as others will ask questions that you may not have thought about but are keen to know the answer.

Please read the parts that are relevant to you at the particular time. Feel free to roam through the various areas and return to some to read again and again. The book is designed to help you understand your part of the partnership. The LAP-BAND™ is highly successful when that partnership is in place. We hope that the book helps you to achieve your share of the safe, gentle and successful weight loss that is unique to the LAP-BAND™.

THE PROBLEM
OF OBESITY

1. Obesity is the most common health problem in our community.

2. Obesity causes many diseases and markedly increases the risk of dying prematurely.

3. Obesity reduces quality of life by limiting physical activity and encouraging social isolation.

4. The costs of obesity through increased health costs and reduced effectiveness in the community are very high.

5. The body mass index or BMI is the best simple method for measuring how obese someone is.

OBESITY IN TODAY'S SOCIETY

Obesity is rapidly becoming one of the greatest health challenges of the 21st century.[1] No disease is more common and causes more unnecessary illness or early death than obesity. Furthermore, there is no other single problem that so reduces the quality of life or increases the demand for health-care services.

The problem is worldwide. In the United States, more than two of every three adults are overweight and about one in three is obese. This means that approximately 60 million people have the disease of obesity in the United States alone. More than one in five Australian adults, an estimated 2.6 million of a population of 20 million, are obese. For both countries, the incidence of obesity has doubled since 1980. Alarmingly, obesity starts in childhood and already 7% of our teenagers are obese.

Around the world, all countries have a growing problem. There are now an estimated 300 million people around the world who are suffering from obesity and its consequences. In both developed and developing nations, a similar pattern is occurring. In Russia, 54% of adults are overweight. In Brazil, the figure is 36%, and in Malaysia, 27%. Even China has a developing problem. A recent survey of adults in urban Shanghai reported that 29.5% were overweight and 4.3% were obese.

After millions of years of evolution we carry a genetic structure designed to enable us to survive the life of the hunter–gatherer, but our health and our lives are now threatened by a lifestyle characterized by ready access to copious amounts of attractive food and very little need for physical activity. Foods high in fat, carbohydrates and, in particular, simple sugars, are booming. The US Department of Agriculture reports that the US per capita intake of sugar was 152.4 lb (69 kg) in 2000. This is equal to nearly half a pound (230 g) of sugar per person each day. Most people will claim that they are not eating that much sugar. However, sugar is now a part of so many foods that we don't even realize that we are eating it. Sugar has infiltrated our diet to a frightening extent. One hundred years ago, the sugar intake per capita was only 0.5 lb (230 g). Is it any wonder that we have a problem with obesity?

And we don't even need to get out of the chair to order the food to be delivered or to change the channels on the television. Activity has become optional. The combination of increased intake of energy and reduced energy expenditure inevitably leads to progressive weight increase.

DEFINING AND MEASURING OBESITY

Obesity is a disease in which fat has accumulated to the extent that health is impaired.

Note that there are three key components to this definition:

1. **"Obesity is a disease ..."** It is only recently that major health authorities such as the World Health Organization and the US Federal Department of Health have acknowledged obesity as a disease. This change is most important as the disease of obesity can now begin to claim attention and an allocation of resources as do all other diseases.

2. **"... in which fat has accumulated ..."** Fat is the key element of obesity. Primarily we are interested in how much fat there is in the body. We are not focused on weight per se. However, as we do not have a simple office method for directly measuring the fat content of the body, we have to use surrogate measures. We could use weight alone but this would be terribly misleading. The tall person is always likely to be heavier than the shorter person. Therefore, as a minimum, we have to take into account the height as well. Currently, our best way to do this is by using the body mass index or the BMI. We will discuss how we calculate the BMI and look at its strengths and weaknesses below.

3. **"... to the extent that health is impaired."** We are
    dealing with a disease that causes disease. The
    disease of obesity may be expressed in various
    ways. It may be as type 2 diabetes or as any of the
    dozens of known diseases that are caused by or made
    worse by obesity. It may be expressed as a physical
    or psychosocial limitation on the quality of your
    life. For example, you can no longer do the things
    that are normally expected. You may have severe
    lowering of self-esteem or self-confidence, leading
    to isolation, depression or unemployment. Or it may
    be expressed as a risk to your future health. You
    may feel fine currently but you are aware that you
    are at high risk of disease in the future and that your
    life expectancy is being reduced by your obesity.

We will look at the disease of obesity in more detail
below but, firstly, let's be clear about how we measure
this disease.

THE BODY MASS INDEX

The BMI is our best single measure of obesity.

The BMI is a measure that combines the weight and
the height according to the following formula:

BMI = weight (in pounds) divided by height^2 (in inches) × 705

  or

BMI = weight (in kilograms) divided by height^2 (in meters)

We use BMI as our primary measure of obesity. We want a measure that is simple to make and acceptably accurate. Direct measure of the amount of fat in the body is not simple and measuring weight alone is not accurate enough. Across the world, the BMI is accepted as the best primary measure because, in most situations, it provides an accurate reflection of the amount of fat present. As weight increases, it is mainly as fat. There may be some increase in muscle mass as well but it is usually small in proportion. As you lose weight, the loss of fat is predominant but you may also lose some muscle mass.

We have now established what we consider are normal and abnormal levels of BMI. The BMI values for Western populations are shown in Table 1.1.

Any level of obesity is bad for you. At a BMI of 30 you are at a higher risk of disease and have a reduced life expectancy. For most, the quality of life is reduced. At progressively higher levels of BMI the likelihood of disease increases, the risk to life is greater and the

TABLE 1.1 BMI VALUES FOR WESTERN POPULATIONS

Label	BMI	Label	BMI
Normal	18.5–25	Severely obese	>35
Overweight	25–30	Morbidly obese	>40
Obese	>30	Super obese	>50

quality of life is less. Of course, there is much variation between individuals. Some people can have quite a high BMI and not recognize any problem. Others can be mildly obese and yet suffer significantly.

If the concept of BMI is confusing to you, Tables 1.2 and 1.3 show the BMI for different weights and heights, in US units and in metric units respectively.

It is important to understand that BMI is not a perfect measure. It is used as a surrogate for measuring the amount of fat. Its great advantage is that it is simple to

TABLE 1.2 BODY MASS INDEX CHART—US UNITS

	Height (in)								
Weight (lb)	60	62	64	66	68	70	72	74	76
120	23	22	21	19	18	17	16	15	15
130	25	24	22	21	20	19	18	17	16
140	27	26	24	23	21	20	19	18	17
150	29	27	26	24	23	22	20	19	18
160	31	29	28	26	24	23	22	21	20
170	33	31	29	27	26	24	23	22	21
180	35	33	31	29	27	26	24	23	22
190	37	35	33	31	29	27	26	24	23
200	39	37	34	32	30	29	27	26	24
210	41	38	36	34	32	30	29	27	26
220	43	40	38	36	34	32	30	28	27
230	45	42	40	37	35	33	31	30	28
240	47	44	41	39	37	35	33	31	29
250	49	46	43	40	38	36	34	32	30
260	51	48	45	42	40	38	36	34	32
270	53	49	46	44	41	39	37	35	33
280	55	51	48	45	43	40	38	36	34
290	57	53	50	47	44	42	39	37	35
300	59	55	52	49	46	43	41	39	37
320	63	59	55	52	48	46	43	41	40
340	66	62	58	55	52	49	46	44	41
360	70	66	62	58	55	52	49	46	44
380	74	70	65	61	58	55	52	49	46
400	78	73	69	65	61	57	54	51	49

TABLE 1.3 BODY MASS INDEX CHART—METRIC UNITS

Weight (kg)	Height (cm)								
	152	158	163	168	173	178	183	188	193
54	23	22	21	19	18	17	16	15	15
59	25	24	22	21	20	19	18	17	16
64	27	26	24	23	21	20	19	18	17
68	29	27	26	24	23	22	20	19	18
73	31	29	28	26	24	23	22	21	20
77	33	31	29	27	26	24	23	22	21
82	35	33	31	29	27	26	24	23	22
86	37	35	33	31	29	27	26	24	23
91	39	37	34	32	30	29	27	26	24
95	41	38	36	34	32	30	29	27	26
100	43	40	38	36	34	32	30	28	27
104	45	42	40	37	35	33	31	30	28
109	47	44	41	39	37	35	33	31	29
113	49	46	43	40	38	36	34	32	30
118	51	48	45	42	40	38	36	34	32
123	53	49	46	44	41	39	37	35	33
127	55	51	48	45	43	40	38	36	34
132	57	53	50	47	44	42	39	37	35
136	59	55	52	49	46	43	41	39	37
145	63	59	55	52	48	46	43	41	40
154	66	62	58	55	52	49	46	44	41
163	70	66	62	58	55	52	49	46	44
172	74	70	65	61	58	55	52	49	46
181	78	73	69	65	61	57	54	51	49

measure and it is generally accurate enough. However, it can be misleading. Below are four examples which demonstrate that BMI is not a perfect measure.

Firstly, the critical cutoff of BMI for obesity is different for some ethnic groups. For people who originated from European countries, the so-called Western world, a BMI of 30 is considered the dividing line between being overweight and obese. But, from careful study of the amount of fat in the body at different weights, we now know that the Chinese, Indian and Malay population should be regarded as obese at BMI levels of 27–28 rather than 30 because at any given weight they will have a higher proportion of fat. As a more detailed picture of the ethnic differences continues to develop we may find other groups who should have different cutoffs also.

Secondly, the athlete who builds up muscle through heavy training can put on weight without additional fat. BMI measures in such a person will not reflect the fat content of the body. There are many examples of bodybuilders or football players who have a high BMI but very little body fat. They do not have obesity as they do not have an abnormal accumulation of fat. As long as we understand that BMI is not a direct but a surrogate measure for fat, we should not get confused by this exception.

Thirdly, the BMI does not tell us anything about the distribution of fat and yet we recognize that those with "central" obesity—the big belly—have a higher risk of a range of obesity-related disorders, such as heart disease and diabetes, compared to those with "peripheral" obesity—big bottom and legs. In other words, the "apple" shape is worse than the "pear" shape. Again, simple observation and measurement enable us to avoid confusion on this.

Finally, the accumulation of excess fat in children and adolescents is not adequately reflected by measuring height and weight alone. We must include age and then look at growth and weight charts to see if the child is outside the expected range.

While we should recognize these potential pitfalls, BMI remains our best general measure. It is used throughout the world, it is easy to measure and to understand, and is now established as the appropriate starting point for describing obesity.

OTHER MEASURES OF FATNESS

Although the BMI is the most commonly used and most simple method for estimating the amount of fat in the body as a proportion of total body weight, we can do this more accurately with some relatively sophisticated tests such as DEXA and underwater weighing.

DEXA
DEXA is now a common test and potentially very useful in measuring fatness and following the fat loss as the weight deceases. DEXA stands for dual energy X-ray absorptiometry. Up to now it has been used mainly for measuring the density of bones

to check for possible thinning of the bones or osteoporosis. The DEXA machine looks a bit like a CT scanner but uses much lower energy and therefore has less potential for harm. It is too complex to use on a day-to-day basis but does tell us exactly how much fat is in the body and can be used intermittently to monitor progress.

UNDERWATER WEIGHING
Underwater weighing is an accurate way to measure the fat content of the body. It provides a simple measure of weight per unit volume and takes us back to Ancient Greece and to Archimedes lying in his bath. He is said to have shouted "eureka" when he realized how, through the displacement of water, he could discover if the King's golden crown contained some base metals. In this same way, we can now discover how much of you is fat. However, although it is accurate and therefore valuable in research studies, it not really acceptable for most people and not suitable for frequent measures.

BIOIMPEDANCE
Bioimpedance, otherwise called BIA, is well known, commonly used and therefore deserves comment. You can readily buy scales that provide measures of bioimpedance and these scales give a readout of total

body fat. You will see them advertised by commercial weight-loss groups, and physicians' offices frequently have them. More complex devices are also available. The concept is that a small electrical current is passed across the body and the resistance to the flow of that current is measured. Fat impedes the flow of the current more than the other body tissues and, from the measurement of this impedance, the instrument uses a formula to calculate how much of the body is fat. Unfortunately, the technique is not an accurate measure of fatness. Because of the way the calculations are performed by these devices, we are able to get just as accurate a measure of the amount of fat by using the BMI alone. Don't be fooled by the fact that it prints out numbers or sounds highly scientific. It is not.

THE PROBLEMS THAT OBESITY CAUSES

1. REDUCED LIFE EXPECTANCY

The first problem of obesity to focus on is the one that many obese people think about the least—you are less likely to live a long life if you are too fat. The life insurance companies have known this for a long time. They know that, for life insurance purposes, the fatter you are the worse the risk you are to them.

The graph in Figure 1.1 shows the risk of dying in a large group of American men and women who were followed for many years. The relative risk of dying is set at 100 for normal weight and the graph shows how your risk increases progressively as you move above a BMI of 27.

If your BMI is greater than 35, you are in the high-risk group and, by the time you reach a BMI of 40, the risk is nearly three times that of people who have normal weight. The risk rises very steeply as your weight goes above a BMI of 40.

FIGURE 1.1 BMI AND THE RISK OF DEATH

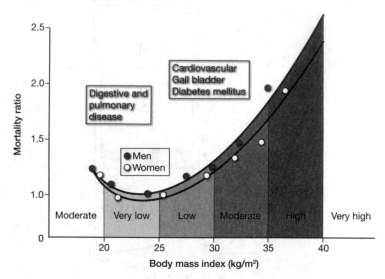

Body mass index (kg/m²)

The Centers for Disease Control in Atlanta, Georgia, estimated that, depending on how you calculate the numbers, there were between 112,000 and 380,000 excess deaths from obesity-related disease in the United States during the year 2000.[2,3] Whichever figure is correct, or something in between, it is an horrific statistic, far worse than road deaths (43,000) or terrorism (0) for that year. Even the young are paying a price for their obesity. Teenagers entering adulthood with a BMI greater than 40 would have their life expectancy reduced by up to 13 years for a male and 8 years for a female. That is a major part of their life lost before they are even adults. The risk of early death from obesity is similar to the risk from smoking.

2. MEDICAL DISEASES

A pathogen is something that causes disease. Obesity is the consummate pathogen. It causes or makes worse a broad range of diseases, such as type 2 diabetes, coronary heart disease and stroke, hypertension, sleep apnea, depression, a range of cancers including breast, gynecological and gastrointestinal malignancies, abnormal levels of fats in the blood, polycystic ovary syndrome, inflammation of the liver, and osteoarthritis of the lower spine and joints that bear your weight, such as the hips, knees and feet.

Also, obese people are more at risk of accidents at work, at home or on the road, and are more likely to suffer sudden unexplained death.

There is a long list of illnesses that are either caused by obesity or are made worse by obesity. The ones that are listed in Table 1.4 are the common and most important of such illnesses.

We will discuss a number of these diseases in Chapter 2 when we will also look at the improvements in health that occur with weight loss. For now we will look at some of the physical, social and economic problems that occur with obesity.

TABLE 1.4 ILLNESSES CAUSED BY OR EXACERBATED BY OBESITY

- Diabetes
- Hypertension
- Dyslipidemia
- Ischemic heart disease
- Cardiomyopathy
- Pulmonary hypertension
- Asthma
- Hypoventilation syndromes
- Obstructive sleep apnea
- Gallstones
- Non-alcoholic steatohepatitis (NASH)
- Urinary incontinence
- Gastroesophageal reflux
- Arthritis—weight bearing

- Low back pain
- Infertility
- Polycystic ovary syndrome
- Obstetric complications
- Deep vein thrombosis (DVT) and thromboembolism
- Depression
- Immobility
- Breast, gastrointestinal, prostate and endometrial cancer
- Venous/stasis ulcers
- Intertrigo
- Accident prone

3. PHYSICAL LIMITATIONS

Morbidly obese people often cannot do the things that others can do. Sporting activities are generally out, which excludes them from many family pastimes. Physical activity of any sort can be quite difficult due to shortness of breath or just plain tiredness, so that even housework or standard employment is a challenge.

Most morbidly obese people cannot buy clothes easily and some have difficulty getting into and out of cars, or into seats on the bus or at the theater.

Airplane travel can be a major embarrassment. You may need to ask for an extension for the seat belt. You may not be able to lower the table down. You may see the person allocated the seat next to you go to the flight attendant and ask for another seat. Just the thought of these things happening can put you off travel.

Flexibility is reduced. The toes get progressively out of reach or even out of sight, making cutting the toenails a shared responsibility. Personal hygiene becomes a problem if you cannot get the toilet paper or the towel to reach all the nooks and crannies.

4. SOCIAL ISOLATION

Many people who are morbidly obese feel uncomfortable in public. Commonly they sense that other people are looking at them and commenting on their weight and the difficulties it produces in dressing well and moving easily. They prefer to withdraw — to live within the family circle at home, rarely venturing into the public gaze.

This may help them cope with the embarrassment but equally it deprives them of the chance to work, to join the family in outside activities and to join friends socially. It is not surprising, therefore, to find that the morbidly obese have a low level of self-esteem and a feeling of worthlessness and uselessness. It is common for obese people to suffer depression. They hate their appearance. They feel that they are unattractive to their partner or children and to others.

Obese people suffer social bias, prejudice and discrimination as a result of their appearance. Society stigmatizes the obesity. Obesity is probably the only area left where discrimination is still considered acceptable. Unfavorable remarks about someone because of their sex, race or disability are not acceptable in our society today, and rightly so. However, unfavorable remarks about someone's obesity are still okay. This attitude is implanted early. When children

My patients are the best witnesses to these problems. The following are a list of anecdotes about events that have occurred to some of them because of their obesity:

1. Waiting in line at the supermarket with a cart of shopping and a stranger will look into the cart and point to items saying "Someone your size shouldn't be eating that."

2. Walking down the street and a small child speaking to her mother in a really loud voice says "Look at that big fat lady. She's the fattest lady I've ever seen." Others all turn to look at me.

3. Walking along the street and a car load of young men/louts yelling obscenities to me about my size.

4. In a nightclub, overhearing a man refer to me as a "beached whale."

5. Traveling in Asia and constantly harassed by locals about my size. There were some very cruel comments and frequent attempts to touch and squeeze parts of my body.

6. At an airport, a very loud and public scene when an official said I was so fat that I had to pay for two seats on the airplane.

7. On an airplane trip I was very publicly moved to another seat as the flight attendant said I was "too heavy and they needed to balance up the weight on the plane."

8. Walking into a dress shop and being told rudely that "there is nothing to fit you here."

9. When shopping I am often totally ignored while other customers receive attention. (This difficulty in clothing shops recurs again and again. And when they have lost weight, they are greeted warmly and asked if they need any help.)

10. Checking that the chairs in a restaurant are strong enough to hold me. They pretend to be anxious that I may break the chair.

11. Getting into an elevator and a woman already inside saying to her child as she looks directly at me, "I think we'll get out here and wait for the next elevator."

are shown the silhouette of an obese person they describe the person as ugly, smelly, dirty, lazy, stupid, dishonest, weak-willed, awkward, a liar and a cheat.

5. ECONOMIC CONSIDERATIONS

Obesity costs the community a great deal in view of the high healthcare needs of the obese.[1] These costs are both the direct costs of investigating and treating obesity-related diseases, such as physician visits, tests, medicines and hospitalizations, and the indirect costs, such as the wages lost because of illness or disability or the loss of future earnings because of premature death. In the United States, these costs were estimated by the US Department of Health and Human Services to be $117 billion for the year 2000. This was made up of $61 billion for direct costs and $56 billion for indirect costs. Major contributors to this total cost are heart disease ($9 billion), osteoarthritis ($21 billion), high blood pressure ($4 billion), gallbladder disease ($3 billion), and cancers of the breast, uterus and colon ($7 billion). Nearly 40 million annual workdays were lost. It was estimated that, in the year 2000 in the United States, people made 63 million visits to their physician because of obesity-related problems.

Whichever way you look at these numbers, we are spending a great deal on obesity. If these costs could be reduced by weight loss, it would pay for a lot of treatments.

SUMMARY

Obesity is truly a problem. It is the worst cause of disease in the Western world. It leads to early death in more people than almost any other cause. What life you do have is severely reduced in quality because of the physical and social problems generated by the disease. And it costs us as a community a great deal of money because of the direct and indirect effects of the health problems. If losing weight solves even some of these problems, and if we can find an acceptable and effective way to lose weight, we really should go for it.

THE BENEFITS OF WEIGHT LOSS

1. Weight loss is the most powerful therapy we have in medicine today.

2. Weight loss from the LAP-BAND™ System leads to the resolution of most of the diseases that arise from obesity.

3. Weight loss from the LAP-BAND™ System improves quality of life.

4. Substantial weight loss after placement of the LAP-BAND™ results in a marked improvement in length of life.

THE POWER OF WEIGHT LOSS

Weight loss is the most powerful therapy we have available in medicine today.

There is no other treatment that can make such a difference to so many health problems. There is no other therapy which improves people's quality of life so much. And, in particular, there is no other therapy that so clearly protects people from dying prematurely.

Chapter 1 highlighted the fact that many diseases are caused by or made worse by obesity. We have seen that obesity reduces the quality of people's lives by limiting them both physically and socially. Also, obesity is rapidly becoming the greatest cause of preventable death, even above smoking. It is natural to assume that, with weight loss, all these problems will go away, that everything will go back to normal and there will be no more trouble. This is not a reasonable assumption to make without some proof.

For instance, obesity could have already resulted in the damage having been done. Although the weight loss might slow the progression of disease, can it really reverse a disease process or improve quality of life after 20 or 30 years of disease? Even with weight loss, people may die just as prematurely, the patient with diabetes may continue to need insulin and the chronically unemployed may still not be able to get work. We need data. If we do not measure it we cannot know. Fortunately, we have now measured most of the problems of obesity and the results are reassuring.

ILLNESSES ASSOCIATED WITH OBESITY

Let's look at the illnesses associated with obesity first. Outlined in boxes are some studies that we have done at the Centre for Obesity Research and Education at Monash University over the last 10 years. All of these studies have been published in the medical literature and are available from a medical library. If you want more detail than the brief summaries provided here, please go to the sources and study the reports in more detail.

TYPE 2 DIABETES

Type 2 diabetes is the paradigm of an obesity-related disease. In most cases, it exists because of obesity and, in most cases, it will disappear with weight loss. It is common, it generates multiple serious complications, and it is lethal.

Most people with type 2 diabetes are overweight and about half are obese. This is particularly well illustrated by the Nurses' Health Study, an important ongoing study in the United States, in which approximately 100,000 nurses have been followed for many years.[4] Based on the risk of developing type 2 diabetes when the BMI is 21, this study showed that the risk of developing type 2 diabetes was five times greater at a BMI of 25, 35 times greater at a BMI of 30, and 93 times greater at or above a BMI of 35. It is estimated that there are now more than 17 million people with type 2 diabetes in the United States and over one million in Australia. Given the morbidity and mortality that diabetes causes in young and middle-aged adults, this disease alone should elicit a very loud call for action against the rising epidemic of obesity.

Most of our patients who were diabetic before LAP-BAND™ placement have either become non-diabetic or have had a significant reduction in the medication they need for control of their sugar levels.

STUDY BOX

We studied 50 patients who had diabetes and severe obesity. At 1 year after LAP-BAND™ placement, 28 (56%) were off all treatment and had normal blood sugar levels and other markers of diabetes. To all intents and purposes they were cured. A further 14 were much improved but still needed some treatment. Thus, a total of 84% had a complete or partial benefit.[5]

No treatment other than weight loss can have such a powerful effect on diabetes. Most treatments strive just to limit the severity and dangers of the disease by keeping the blood sugar levels as near to normal as possible. Weight loss can take the disease away completely. Diabetes is a dreadful disease. It damages most systems of the body and severely shortens life expectancy. Weight loss can change the disease dramatically. If you are obese and have type 2 diabetes, it is essential that you lose weight. This should be seen as the most important part of the treatment of diabetes. If the simpler options of lifestyle change through less eating and more exercise have not succeeded, LAP-BAND™ placement must be considered.

HYPERTENSION

High blood pressure is a major risk factor for heart attacks and strokes. It is much more common in the obese.

STUDY BOX

We followed 88 people with high blood pressure for 12 months after LAP-BAND™ placement and found that, by that time, 60% had returned to normal blood pressure and were off all treatment. Another 33% had found their blood pressure was much easier to control.[6]

ABNORMAL FATS IN THE BLOOD

Medically we call this problem dyslipidemia—"dys" means disordered, "lipid" is another word for fat and "emia" refers to the blood. In obese people the triglyceride levels are often elevated and, the high-density lipoprotein (HDL) cholesterol, which is sometimes referred to as the "good" cholesterol, is abnormally low.

STUDY BOX

We have followed several hundred patients for 4 years after LAP-BAND™ placement and have found that the triglyceride and HDL cholesterol levels rapidly return to normal and stay there for at least the 4 years. As abnormalities of these lipid levels is a clear risk factor for heart disease, this reduction in levels is regarded as very beneficial.[7]

REFLUX ESOPHAGITIS

This problem is sometimes referred to as GERD, an abbreviation for gastroesophageal reflux disease. It is very common in the obese. More than half the people we see with severe obesity have some heartburn. This is the pain or uncomfortable feeling you get behind the breastbone when acid from the stomach travels up into the esophagus and irritates the lining enough to give symptoms. About one in five of our patients will have this problem severely enough to have to take drug therapy to reduce the acid. If the disease continues for long enough, a change, known as Barrett's esophagus, can occur in the lining of the esophagus. This new lining is regarded as premalignant. It carries a 50 times increase in the chance of developing cancer of the esophagus.

More than half our patients have heartburn before the LAP-BAND™ placement and almost all are cured by the procedure.

STUDY BOX

We followed 88 patients who had a moderate or severe stage of GERD. At 12 months 90% had no further symptoms and were not taking any medication for the problem.[8]

The LAP-BAND™ is very good at blocking reflux. This is a direct effect of the band sitting at the very top of the stomach, where it can stop the acid moving up into the esophagus. The benefit is felt immediately after operation, before any weight loss has had time to occur. We have had a lot of experience with the operation of Nissen fundoplication. This is a laparoscopic operation that is very good for controlling GERD in the general population. Our results with LAP-BAND™ placement are just as good as are our results with Nissen fundoplication. For someone who has severe GERD and severe obesity, two problems are solved for the price of one.

SLEEP-DISORDERED BREATHING

The most significant disorder of breathing while asleep is obstructive sleep apnea and we will look at this problem below. Other breathing problems include habitual snoring, daytime sleepiness and poor sleep quality.

STUDY BOX

We looked at 313 of our obese patients before LAP-BAND™ placement and found that 59% of the men and 45% of the women had some form of disturbed sleep. We restudied 123 of these people at 1 year after band placement, by which time they had lost nearly half of their excess weight. The habitual snoring had decreased from 82% to 14% of patients, abnormal daytime sleepiness was reduced from 40% to 4% patients, and poor sleep quality was reduced from 40% to 2% of patients. As a group they were snoring less, sleeping better and felt less tired during the day.[9]

We were a little surprised to find that the problems were nearly as common in the women as the men and yet the men are much more likely to attract medical attention and have proper sleep assessments performed.

OBSTRUCTIVE SLEEP APNEA

Obstructive sleep apnea (OSA) is a disease in which you stop breathing during your sleep. The word "apnea" means "no breathing." Typically, you are snoring away as usual and then there is a period of quiet. Your partner is delighted for the moment of peace and quiet but anxious that there is absolutely no sound. You could be dead. There may be silence for up to a minute. Then, with a lot of grunts and snorts, you get going again back to heavy snoring.

What has happened is that the tissues in the neck have become too bulky and there is inadequate space. As you start to go into the deep phase of sleep, your muscles relax, and your tongue falls back and closes the small space present, blocking your airway. As the oxygen levels in the body fall, the brain stirs, wakes you up and tells you to get back to some serious breathing. You wake up, get some tone back in the tongue, the airway opens and the snoring show is back on the road. These episodes may happen 100 times a night. They are not good for the brain or the heart—or the marriage. You don't get a good night's sleep and are drowsy through the day. The drowsy driver is now recognized as a major contributor to road deaths. It is bad for you and dangerous for others.

In the study of sleep-disordered breathing described above, we found that one-third of the patients had observed sleep apnea before LAP-BAND™ placement. By that we mean that their partner observed them stopping breathing during periods of heavy snoring. After weight loss, only 2% had the problem.

STUDY BOX

In a later study we examined sleep apnea more closely by doing sleep studies before and at an average of 18 months after LAP-BAND™ placement. In the sleep study, each person has their sleep status and their breathing monitored overnight in a sleep laboratory. We studied 25 men and women who were massively obese with an average BMI of 53. Before operation, 23 had been diagnosed as having sleep apnea and were using continuous positive airway pressure (CPAP) machines to help them through the night. The other two had sleep apnea but were not using CPAP. After an average weight loss of 99 lb (45 kg) each, only six were still using their CPAP machines and all of those machines were set at lower pressures. As a group they also noticed a major improvement in other health measures, improved quality of life, less depression and less daytime sleepiness. The health benefits of weight loss for these people were very clear. And the pleasure of being able to go to bed at night without the mask and the machine was very gratefully received.[10]

ASTHMA

Asthma has only recently been recognized as an important illness associated with obesity. It is at least twice as common in obese children and adults as those with normal weight. Weight loss as a result of LAP-BAND™ placement has helped almost every one of our asthmatic patients. All find it easier to manage their asthma and to avoid severe attacks, and some have no more trouble with asthma after they have lost weight. In our studies we found a remarkable reduction in the need to be admitted to hospital for asthma. All patients who have asthma will show an improvement in association with weight loss after band placement. In some cases, there will be no further attacks and no need for continuing therapy.

STUDY BOX

In a specific study of the effects of weight loss on asthma, we followed 33 patients for 1 year. All showed improvement with less attacks and easier control. One-third of the patients had no asthma attacks at all during the year. In the year before the LAP-BAND™ procedure nine of the group had required admission to hospital on one or more occasions because of acute episodes of asthma. No admissions to hospital were needed in the year after operation.[11]

NON-ALCOHOLIC STEATOHEPATITIS (NASH)

This name is a bit of a mouthful but simply means inflammation of the liver ("hepatitis") associated with fat ("steato") and not due to excess alcohol consumption. The acronym NASH is easier to use. NASH occurs particularly in obese people who have a lot of their weight in the middle—the apple-shaped—and who are at risk of diabetes or already have diabetes. You may not have heard much about it but it is becoming recognized as a major health problem and is now one of the common diseases leading to the need for a liver transplant. If we think you are at risk of NASH, we will take a biopsy of the liver at the time of LAP-BAND™ placement to check for it.

STUDY BOX

We have studied 36 patients who had a liver biopsy at the time of LAP-BAND™ placement and then we took a second liver biopsy at approximately 2 years after band placement to check if the problem was resolving with weight loss. NASH was present at the initial biopsy in 23 of these patients but was present in only four of these people at repeat biopsy. The changes associated with weight loss had led to resolution of this dangerous condition in 19 of the 23 people.[12]

INFERTILITY AND POLYCYSTIC OVARY SYNDROME

Obesity leads to infertility in women most commonly due to irregular ovulation or no ovulation at all. One particular condition that is common in obese women is polycystic ovary syndrome, often abbreviated to PCOS. In this condition there are abnormalities that lead to an excess of the male hormone, testosterone, in the circulation. Many of these women notice acne and excess hair on the face in association with very irregular periods. Weight loss leads to correction of the hormonal problems, so that periods become more regular and fertility increases.

STUDY BOX

In a study of the hormonal changes in 107 obese women, 12 were shown to have PCOS initially. This resolved in 11 of the 12 as they lost weight.[13]

PREGNANCY

Not only are women more likely to become pregnant after losing weight, they will also have a better outcome. Pregnancy in severely obese women is associated with important risks to both the mother and the baby. Do women who have lost weight after LAP-BAND™ placement have less problems?

STUDY BOX

Over 100 pregnancies have occurred in our patients after LAP-BAND™ placement. We compared these pregnancy outcomes with those of the pregnancies they had before band placement and with the outcomes of pregnancy that we have come to expect in the general community.

After band placement the pregnant women did just fine. The weight gained during the pregnancy was about the right amount—16–19 lb (7–9 kg). This was because of a very important asset of the LAP-BAND™—its adjustability. We can remove fluid if the weight gain is not ideal and allow a greater food intake, enough for the pregnant mother and the growing baby. Other bariatric procedures do not allow this margin of nutritional safety.

The birth weights of the babies were identical to those in the general community—about 7 lb (3.3 kg)—and there was about the same incidence of problems such as high blood pressure, diabetes and need for caesarian section as occur in the general community. These outcomes were clearly better than had occurred in the previous pregnancies of these women before they had lost the weight.[14]

DEPRESSION

Depression is common in obese people.

STUDY BOX

We followed the outcome of 262 consecutive patients with LAP-BAND™ placement. We measured their level of depression before operation and found that they were almost equally divided into four groups. Approximately one-quarter were not depressed at all, and one-quarter each had mild depression, moderate depression or severe depression. We followed them for up to 4 years and noticed a major and durable improvement. At the end of the study three out of four were judged to be not depressed and very few were left with moderate or severe depression.[15]

OTHER BENEFITS OF WEIGHT LOSS

THE EFFECTS OF WEIGHT LOSS ON SURVIVAL

We all want to live a long life. We don't want to die prematurely. It is clear that obesity is associated with a reduced life expectancy due to the effects of all the diseases it causes. Heart disease, stroke, cancers and all the complications of diabetes are just some of the dangerous problems that could lead to early death. But do you live longer if you have been obese and lose weight?

STUDY BOX

We have been seeking the answer to this question by looking at the outcomes for our patients who have lost weight after LAP-BAND™ placement and comparing the number of deaths that have occurred in our patients with an equivalent group of people who were obese but have not lost weight. In summary, we have followed 1466 patients for an average of 3.6 years and compared them to a group of 2119 obese patients who remained obese and who were followed for an average of 12 years. There have been no deaths in our patients from the band placement itself but five patients have died from causes such as heart attack and cancer in the years after surgery. A total of 225 have died in the group who have not lost weight. Once we adjust for the different length of follow-up, age, sex and weight differences, the risk of dying has been reduced in the LAP-BAND™ group by 73%. The obese group had four times the risk of dying during the follow-up period compared to the group who lost weight after band placement.

This is a very powerful effect. Hopefully it will cause the healthcare providers and administrators to take notice of the potential benefits of the LAP-BAND™ System and be more enthusiastic about funding the procedure. We often hear in the press about another "breakthrough" in medicine when a new treatment is able to achieve a 20% improvement in survival over the existing treatment. In this case there is a 400% increase, making LAP-BAND™ placement 20 times more powerful than some of the other breakthroughs noted in medicine.

QUALITY OF LIFE

Obesity has a major impact on the physical, psychosocial and economic health of patients and thus we could expect that it reduces the quality of life. But how can we know? How can we measure quality of life? Fortunately, there are now quite a number of ways of doing this which are easy to do and have been shown to be valid measures. The most broadly accepted is a set of 36 questions known as the Medical Short Form (36) Health Survey or, more briefly, the SF-36. This questionnaire can measure quality of life across a range of health conditions.

STUDY BOX

We have used the SF-36 to assess the quality of life in obese people and the changes that occur with weight loss after LAP-BAND™ placement. In one study we tested 459 patients before operation and then annually for 4 years. In the obese people all measures of the SF-36 were significantly lower than in the general community, indicating a markedly reduced quality of life. The values were equivalent to the reduced quality of life that can be measured in people with extensive cancer, crippling arthritis or stroke. At the end of the first year after band placement, all measures had returned to the normal values for the community as a whole and they remained so for the 4 years of the study.[16]

However, perhaps the best demonstration of the improvement in quality of life comes not from the dry science of our research but from the stories our patients tell us about the simple pleasures they recognize after weight loss:

---

1. being able to cross your legs when sitting

2. spending all day in the garden without having to stop every 15 minutes

3. not being the fattest person in the room

4. buying clothes off the rack

5. not having to take several prescription drugs every day

6. being confident enough to apply for a job and look forward to the interview

7. not being scared of trying on clothes when the label says "one size fits all"

8. going into good clothing shops and being offered assistance instead of being ignored

9. being able to buy a pair of jeans

10. having more self-confidence

11. going out to dinner and ordering an appetizer only, knowing that it will be more than enough

12. looking forward to going to a party

13. being able to get in and out of a car easily

14. climbing a flight of stairs without getting winded

15. having acquaintances say to you "I heard you speak and knew it was your voice but I didn't recognize you"

16. getting outside and involved in the kids' activities

17. having your husband say how good you look and when he looks at photos of the "old" you, says that he can't remember you looking the way you did

18. forgetting you have not eaten

19. no longer dreading the school reunion

20. not thinking about food

21. having the odd food treat and not feeling guilty

22. being able to walk for hours without chafing

23. being able to do up the seat belt on an airplane without the embarrassment of having to ask for an extension

24. feeling energized

25. enjoying moving—springing out of the chair instead of levering yourself out

26. playing sport again

27. keeping up with people walking, especially my husband who takes big strides

28. sitting on the floor, cross-legged

29. dancing; no longer being the fat one in the corner

30. getting down on the floor to play with the kids

31. knowing that my health has improved and that my life has been extended.

SUMMARY

These studies are provided to give you a summary of the remarkable health benefits that have occurred for our patients after LAP-BAND™ placement. These results have all been published or are about to be published in the medical literature after careful scrutiny by experts. As a part of our commitment to keep in touch, we track our patients very carefully and are especially interested in the health benefits that are achieved. Substantial weight loss, as occurs after LAP-BAND™ placement, is the most powerful therapy we have in healthcare today. There is no drug or operation or other treatment that is close to the effectiveness of weight loss on a person with the disease of obesity and its associated illnesses. To have a gentle, safe and reliable way of achieving this weight loss, through LAP-BAND™ placement, is a great joy to us and a great benefit to our patients.

THE OPTIONS FOR ACHIEVING WEIGHT LOSS

1. We must continue to seek preventive measures but these are not available yet.

2. The general expectations of what should be achieved and what needs to be avoided should be established before looking at the different options.

3. Always begin with the simple and safe procedures, and then move to the more complex and risky.

4. Non-surgical options are not yet effective enough for treating obesity.

5. The surgical options are all effective but vary in risk and change to the anatomy.

WAYS TO ACHIEVE WEIGHT LOSS

We have seen that obesity is a major problem and that weight loss is the most powerful therapy we have in healthcare today. It is now time to look at the ways available for achieving this weight loss.

PREVENTION

Firstly, we must mention prevention. This has to be the most important aim to seek.

With a problem so common, there is no way that we can ever treat all those who are or will become obese. We must try to prevent the problem arising in the first place. This has to be our first commitment, particularly to our children and adolescents.

We talk about primary prevention and secondary prevention. By primary prevention we mean avoiding obesity ever occurring. By secondary prevention we mean prevention of the diseases that can arise from obesity, even if we have not been able to prevent obesity itself from occurring.

Unfortunately, at this stage, we are not very good at primary prevention. We have no successful programs that can be applied across our community to prevent the problem of obesity occurring. We have a lot of good ideas, plenty of theories and hypotheses. We even have some pilot studies that may show promise. But, to date, we have no proven, predictable way of prevention that is acceptable to the community and effective in preventing weight gain.

This is not all that surprising. We live in a culture, reinforced by powerful commercial forces, that promotes eating and physical inactivity. To address this established culture will take a strong political will and a multidisciplinary approach. This has not yet happened. We need to continue to look for good pathways to prevention but they are not yet visible. Not only is the problem of obesity still a problem, it is in fact getting worse. The numbers are increasing. We are losing ground. We are visibly failing to prevent the problem. We have not yet even started to overcome this challenge.

We are a little better at secondary prevention. If you develop type 2 diabetes, we can help you control your blood sugar levels and so prevent some of the complications of the disease. If your blood pressure is too high or the fat levels in your blood are too high, we can give you medicines that help control these problems and thereby reduce the chance of stroke or heart attack. However, this is a compromise. You still have the disease and the medicines are just reducing some of its harmful effects but they are not taking it away, nor curing it. It would be far better to get rid of the disease altogether. With significant and durable weight loss, type 2 diabetes can go away, blood pressure can return to normal levels and the fat levels in the blood can return to normal. Most of the obesity-related diseases are either cured or markedly improved with weight loss. Naturally this is our preferred approach, so let us look at methods for achieving weight loss and, in doing so, it should become clear why the LAP-BAND™ is our preferred option for those who have failed the simpler methods.

ACHIEVABLE EXPECTATIONS

Before looking at each of the options for reducing weight we should establish some general expectations of what we want to achieve and at what cost. We can then look at each option and measure its effect against these expectations.

WHAT SHOULD BE REQUIRED FOR ALL TREATMENT OPTIONS?

1. SAFETY
Beyond all else we must try to avoid hurting people. Everything has possible side effects and complications. These need to be minimal. The method you

select to lose weight is a choice you make. It is the balance between the good—the effectiveness—and the bad—the risks and the costs. The good should always far exceed the bad.

2. EFFECTIVENESS

The treatment option should be effective in achieving sufficient weight loss to solve your problem. If you are overweight, a small weight loss might suffice. If you are obese (BMI > 30) you are more likely to need a substantial weight loss to solve your problems. Depending on your initial weight and BMI, a loss of 45–260 lb (20–120 kg) might be needed. Certainly, 11–22 lb (5–10 kg) is not going to be enough. Along with the weight loss, you should also check that there is good evidence of health benefits and a better quality of life with the treatment option.

3. DURABILITY

There is no particular value in short-term weight loss. In fact, there may even be harm. Losing weight, even quite substantial amounts of weight, is not so hard. Most of our patients have done it many times before they come to see us. The real challenge is to keep that weight off for a long time. We, therefore, should look not only at the amount of weight a treatment can achieve but also for evidence that the weight loss lasts.

4. MINIMAL SIDE EFFECTS

Being obese is unpleasant but you don't want to swap one type of unpleasantness for another. If a treatment creates its own problems, such as the oily rectal incontinence that results from taking orlistat or the smelly diarrhea from biliopancreatic diversion, it is not much fun. Check beforehand as to what are the possible side effects of each treatment.

5. CONTROLLABLE/ADJUSTABLE

Lifestyle methods are controllable or adjustable as you can control the amount you eat or the exercise you do. There is also some flexibility with the doses of drugs used for weight loss. For all surgical procedures, except the LAP-BAND™, you do not have this ability. In the future there will be more options that are adjustable but these are not available at this stage. Once the surgeon has left the operating room after a gastric bypass, there is nothing that can be done to vary the restriction created. If it's too tight, bad luck. If it's too loose, too bad. If it's just right, it may slowly alter over time and you or your physician cannot take it back to where it was without difficult surgery.

Having control is very important. Good weight loss programs center on a partnership between you and your physician or other health professional. You both need to be able to exercise some control of the treatment to optimize the effect. Without doubt, the adjustability of the LAP-BAND™ is its greatest single asset—it allows you to control your level of satiety.

6. REVERSIBILITY

We can easily stop a diet or a course of drug treatment. We can remove an intragastric balloon. However, for surgical procedures, the LAP-BAND™ is the only one that is easily reversible. Reversibility is almost as important as adjustability for two reasons. Firstly, we all are skeptical. We worry that something promised may not turn out just so. You do not want to be trapped into something that may not turn out to be what you expected. With the LAP-BAND™, you are not trapped in a permanent state. It can be removed easily and everything goes back to normal. However, this is not so with other surgical procedures—they are there for life.

The second reason to look for reversibility is that we can only look into the future so far. At the moment there is nothing better than the LAP-BAND™ in view. However, in 20 years time, maybe even in 15 years, there could be a dramatically better treatment discovered. You don't want to be locked into something that is well past its use-by date. You want to be able to choose the best current option.

If, however, in the meantime, you have gone ahead with the LAP-BAND™, you can at least be comforted that, if some magical new therapy does arise which works superbly and has minimal side effects, you can have the band removed as a day procedure, the stomach can return to normal and you can start on the new "magical" treatment. The LAP-BAND™ is fully reversible.

Not so if you have had a gastric bypass. This is very difficult procedure to reverse as the stomach has been divided completely and the intestines have been dramatically rearranged. For most of these patients, there can be no going back.

7. LOW REOPERATION/REVISION RATE
Naturally, you would like to have one procedure and that will be all. Unfortunately, this does not always happen. Something may change or leak or block or break, and thus may lead to the need for additional procedures. There is a maintenance requirement for each of the surgical procedures. You need to be aware how likely reoperation is and how complex and risky is the revision.

8. MINIMALLY INVASIVE
If you are going to have surgery, you will want to have as little trauma and changes to your gut as possible. Look for the procedure that interferes with the tissues the least. Ask about what is done for each procedure.

Are organs or parts of them removed? Are segments of the gut closed off or redirected? Is there joining of one part of the gut to another? Remember, leaks from these joins are the major cause of deaths in patients who undergo surgery.

THE TREATMENT OPTIONS

We will now review the options available. The first step in solving your problem with obesity is to make a commitment to lose weight. Lock onto that commitment and accept that your problem is too bad and too dangerous to continue with. The second step is to determine how to do this. There are a series of treatment options and you should start with the simplest and safest before moving on to the more complex and risky. If you are truly committed to losing weight, somewhere along that series you will find the correct option for you. It does require that commitment. You cannot just go part of the way and then give up. You must stay committed.

The list of desirable features above should help you find the right option. We will return to this list after we have looked at the different treatment options to see the strengths and the weaknesses of each. Keep this list of features in mind as we look at each of the treatment options and see what it has to offer. See Table 4.1 for a list of how well each treatment option fulfills the ideal.

1. LIFESTYLE

The lifestyle solution is to eat less food and have plenty of activity. This solution is simple to prescribe yet very difficult to achieve sustainable outcomes. Across the world and across generations a healthy lifestyle through good eating and exercise practices has been constantly promoted; yet the problem of obesity is not just continuing but increasing.

Almost everyone can lose some weight through a diet or exercise program. The challenge is to lose enough weight to make a difference and, more importantly, to keep it off. Weight loss for 1 or 2 years is not much help to your health. You need to lose weight permanently. Very few will lose weight through lifestyle change alone and be able to keep that weight off for even 5 years.

The commercial weight-loss centers have made fortunes by promising excellent weight loss through various twists on the "lifestyle" methods, and their constant advertisements always show the classic "before and after" pictures. Invariably, the "after" picture is only months after. They do not show the "after" pictures at 5 years.

A recent comprehensive review of all the high-quality scientific studies of the options for weight control has found that there is no evidence of a durable effect from any current lifestyle intervention methods for obesity.[17] We would hope that lifestyle approaches could at least prevent the problem. This has not yet been achieved. The problem is increasing. If we are failing to prevent it, we must have less hope of curing it once it is established. The results are therefore not surprising.

VERY-LOW-CALORIE DIET

One particular form of dietary therapy that can have a powerful effect in the short term is the very-low-calorie diet (VLCD). The best known form of the VLCD is called Optifast. This involves taking three sachets of a specially formulated powder each day and almost no other food. Each sachet is made up into a liquid meal with water. You are allowed a small amount of vegetables at night as the only additional intake. If you follow the rules completely you will be receiving between 500 and 600 calories (2100 and 2520 kJ) per day and you may lose 33–66 lb (15–30 kg) over a 3-month period. It is not recommended that you continue beyond 3 months and it is uncommon to succeed so well with a second course later on.

However, you can get good weight loss in the short term. The VLCD provides perhaps our best method for achieving a significant weight loss quickly without resorting to weight loss surgery. There can be reasons why this is a good idea. A common one is as a preparation for a surgical procedure such as a knee or hip operation. We frequently use the VLCD in some patients as a preparation for the LAP-BAND™ procedure, particularly if they have severe central obesity. As it is not continued permanently, you cannot expect to achieve a medium- or long-term weight loss with the VLCD.

2. DRUG THERAPY

We do not yet have drugs that are truly effective for treating obesity. Two drugs are currently available for long-term use for achieving and maintaining weight loss—orlistat (sold as Xenical) and sibutramine (sold as Meridia or Reductil). Both are able to help treat people who are overweight but neither has proven to be sufficiently powerful to be reliable for treating people with obesity. The long-term efficacy is poor and the long-term safety is unknown. A review of all the clinical trials of these drugs shows that the average weight loss after 1 year of orlistat is about 7 lb (3 kg) and for sibutramine is 10 lb (4.5 kg).[18] For those with obesity, who must lose 50 lb (23 kg) or more, these results are just not good enough.

New drugs appear on the horizon frequently and some of these do get into clinical practice. The latest to attract serious interest is rimonabant. In a recent clinical trial this drug produced an average weight loss of 15 lb (6.8 kg) at 12 months.[19] This is still not enough to cure obesity but it is of potential for those who are overweight. It will probably appear on the market in 2007 and will give the community a high expectation for a while.

Most of our patients have tried some of the drug therapies before considering the LAP-BAND™. Anything may be worth a try if the problems of obesity can be overcome. However, it is best not to expect too much—they are not that good. Furthermore, they are usually expensive, they may have unpleasant or even serious side effects, and the thought of taking one of these drugs every day for years and years in order to get a few pounds of weight off is just not acceptable to most people, especially when so little weight loss is achieved.

We definitely need better drugs for obesity. No doubt they will come. We may one day find a pill that truly takes away your appetite, or increases the wasting of energy. There may be some gene therapy that makes you thin forever. The pharmaceutical companies are working very hard to find such drugs or treatments. Given that there is nothing that is dramatically good on the horizon and that it would take 5–10 years from development to market, we probably should not anticipate success from drug therapy in the next 15 years and possibly not in the next 20 years.

3. ENDOSCOPIC PROCEDURES

Endoscopic procedures are those whereby a gastroscope, which is a long flexible tube of light fibers, optical fibers and other channels, is passed through the mouth, down the esophagus and into the stomach. These procedures have not yet established a role in the treatment of obesity but there is plenty of effort seeking an effective method.

Intragastric balloons are the only endoscopic method which is currently in clinical practice around the world. With this method, an empty balloon is passed through the mouth into the stomach. It is then filled with about a pint (0.5 L) of saline and thereby creates a large mass in the stomach. The idea is that you feel full and do not eat so much. After 6 months, the balloon must be removed as it may rupture and cause a blockage further down the gut.

Intragastric balloons were used enthusiastically in the 1980s until carefully performed clinical trials showed them to be ineffective. A new version of the intragastric balloon, the BioEnterics Intragastric Balloon™, commonly known as the BIB™, has been developed with the proposal that it overcomes all the weaknesses of the earlier balloons. It is being used extensively in Europe, Mexico and South America. It is approved for clinical use in Australia but not yet in the United States.

In the clinical reports available the BIB™ appears to work but has yet to demonstrate effectiveness in high-quality clinical trials. It can be left in place for only 6 months, during which time there may be a weight loss of 35 lb (16 kg) or more. The lost weight is likely to return after its removal. Nevertheless, it does appear to make a difference, it does not involve an operation and it is reversible.

There is a high level of research activity seeking other ways of achieving weight loss by methods involving endoscopic techniques. These include ways of suturing or stapling the stomach through the endoscope to simulate what is done in some surgical procedures. It is likely that some of these procedures will appear soon and be publicized as the ultimate solution. It is even more likely that their benefit will, in fact, be modest and short term. We just have to wait and see what happens.

4. WEIGHT LOSS (BARIATRIC) SURGERY

The surgical treatment of obesity is called bariatric surgery after the Greek words, *baros*, meaning "weight," and *iatrikos*, meaning "the art of healing." This is the most rapidly growing area of surgical practice in the Western world today. This reflects the ability of bariatric surgical procedures to provide a solution to an otherwise insoluble problem and the evolution of safer, less invasive and more conservative forms of procedures.

The surgical treatment of obesity has evolved over a period of more than 50 years. Today there are three bariatric procedures in use: gastric bypass, biliopancreatic diversion and laparoscopic adjustable gastric banding. Small bowel bypass is no longer performed.

SMALL BOWEL BYPASS

This procedure was introduced in the 1950s and there were various ways in which this operation was performed. Each method, however, shared the common principle of bypassing the normal absorptive capacity of the gut. In other words, you could eat quite a lot but the food wouldn't be absorbed into the body. Instead, you would have diarrhea. Such procedures were generally effective in achieving weight loss but they had a number of serious side effects, which ultimately has made them unacceptable.

GASTRIC BYPASS

This operation was introduced more than 35 years ago and is still a good procedure. However, it does require major manipulation of the gut. Gastric bypass is most commonly used in the United States and about half of the operations are performed by the traditional open surgical approach with a long incision in the abdomen and half are performed laparoscopically (keyhole surgery).

The operation can be performed in a number of different ways but they all achieve their effect through two common features. Firstly, they create a small upper stomach so that you can only eat a small amount of food at any one time before you feel comfortably or uncomfortably full. Secondly, they each delay the emptying of the food from that small upper stomach into the rest of the gut in some way so that the feeling of fullness stays with you after the meal and you are not inclined to eat between meals.

In gastric bypass procedures, a stapling device is used to cut and separate completely a small piece of the top of the stomach from the rest of the stomach. The top part becomes the new stomach and the rest is closed off and not accessible any more. The upper part of the small intestine is then divided completely, again with the stapling device. One of the divided ends is attached to the new stomach to allow the food to enter the rest of the gut. The other end is joined to the small intestine further downstream so that the digestive juices from the liver, gallbladder, duodenum and pancreas can get back into the digestive pathway. Figure 3.1 shows the end result of these multiple changes.

FIGURE 3.1 GASTRIC BYPASS PROCEDURE

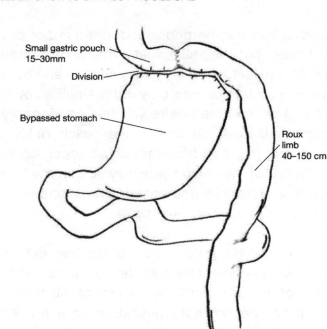

Stomach stapling is a big operation with a real risk of major complications and approximately 1% of people die from these complications. It causes major changes in the gut and is essentially irreversible. The most common form of stomach stapling now used is the Roux-en-Y gastric bypass. This can be done as an open operation or laparoscopically. It is a relatively complex procedure that provides no opportunity for adjustment after the operation.

Another form of gastric stapling that is becoming more commonly used at some centers is the sleeve gastrectomy, in which most of the stomach is removed and discarded and a thin tube is left, with the hope that it will not expand in the years to come. Our previous experience strongly suggests that hope will not be realized. So far there has been very little published information about this procedure. We currently don't know about its risks and benefits and we don't know if the weight loss effect will last for even 5 years.

BILIOPANCREATIC DIVERSION

Biliopancreatic diversion, commonly abbreviated to BPD, was introduced in the 1970s. This complex procedure removes much of the stomach and bypasses much of the gut. This procedure aims to reduce the size of the stomach to restrict intake and also to prevent absorption of the food by diverting it from the digestive enzymes of the gut. Although it can be done laparoscopically, it is generally performed through an abdominal incision to reduce the risks. About half to three-quarters of the stomach is removed completely. The small intestine is then divided and reconnected in such a way that the food goes one way (the alimentary

FIGURE 3.2 BILIOPANCREATIC DIVERSION

Proximal stomach
200–500 mL

Biliopancreatic limb

Alimentary limb
200 cm

Common
channel
50 cm

limb) and the digestive enzymes go another way (the biliopancreatic limb). Most of the enzymes are reabsorbed before they can do anything. The rest of the enzymes meet the food in the last 2 feet (50 cm) of the small intestine—the common channel—to permit some limited absorption of food.

A variation of the BPD is known as the duodenal switch. It differs in only a minor way by changing the way most of the stomach is removed to retain the lower part of the stomach. It is not clear that there is any important difference between the two procedures. The BPD generally achieves good weight loss but at the cost of significant symptoms and a serious risk of malnutrition, and so is not often performed. It can be done as an open operation or, sometimes, laparoscopically. It has the highest likelihood of death associated with the surgery of all the bariatric procedures.

LAPAROSCOPIC ADJUSTABLE GASTRIC BANDING
The LAP-BAND™ is an example of laparoscopic adjustable gastric banding and has been available since the 1990s. LAP-BAND™ placement is far more gentle and safer than the preceding operations. It is almost always done laparoscopically (keyhole surgery) and it involves very little handling or dissection of the tissues. Nothing is cut or stapled or removed or redirected. The band is placed across the very top of the stomach.

There is almost no stomach above the band. With minimal dissection a pathway is made across the back of the top of the stomach, and the band is placed along that pathway, closed and fixed into that position by suturing some of the stomach wall across the front of the band. The tubing is then connected to an access port which is placed under the skin of the abdominal wall.

FIGURE 3.3 LAPAROSCOPIC ADJUSTABLE GASTRIC BANDING PROCEDURE

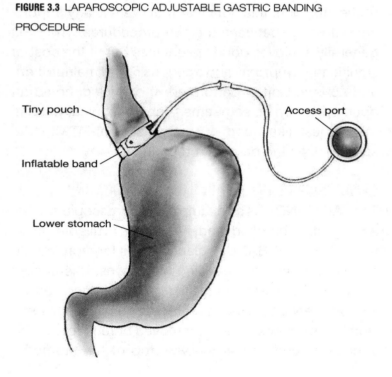

Tiny pouch

Access port

Inflatable band

Lower stomach

WHICH PROCEDURE IS THE MOST COMMON?

There is significant variation in the preferred procedure between countries, often reflecting local regulatory and insurance factors.

In the United States, gastric bypass is still the most common option. The LAP-BAND™ did not become available in the United States until 2001 and many insurance groups are still trying to avoid offering this option to their participants. However, the number of bands placed is increasing rapidly and is expected to become much more common than the gastric bypass option.

In Australia, the LAP-BAND™ is the procedure of choice for more than 90% of people, with gastric bypass making up most of the rest of the procedures.

Biliopancreatic diversion is an uncommon procedure everywhere because of the risks, the constant presence of an offensive diarrhea and the concerns about the effects that a long-term lack of key nutrients will have on the body. In many countries it is not used at all.

COMPARISON OF PROCEDURES

At their best, gastric bypass and the other stomach stapling procedures are very good, enabling a good weight loss without too many side effects. However, they are not at their best often enough. The real dilemma with stomach stapling is how to create a new stomach that is exactly right on the day of operation and which remains exactly right for the rest of the patient's life. This challenge is obviously too difficult. The body will always be changing, particularly stretching, in response to pressure.

Sometimes the settings are too tight initially, resulting in severe vomiting. At other times the settings are too loose, with insufficient weight loss. Most commonly, the settings are about right at the time of operation, but change over subsequent months and years so that, with stretching or with breakdown of the staple line, there is a return toward a normal stomach and the weight-reducing effect is lost.

The best weight loss after gastric bypass is in the first year. Generally, if you have not lost enough weight by then, you are not going to lose any more. The weight starts to come back on again after the second or third year. Because there is no ability to adjust the settings after the operation, the weight regain is not able to be controlled. It is very difficult for us to be sure about how durable the weight loss is after gastric bypass because more than half the people who have the operation are lost to follow-up by 5 years and so we cannot measure their weight. For those that are still being seen, it is most commonly reported that they have lost between 50% and 60% of their excess weight. If we assume that the ones who are missing have done less well—the usual reason why people stop coming to follow-up—the weight loss is probably well under 50% of excess weight at 10 years. This is not as good as has been achieved with the LAP-BAND™.

STUDY BOX

We performed a very thorough analysis of the medical literature bringing together all the reports on gastric bypass and all the reports on LAP-BAND™ placement. We carefully analyzed the data from these reports and created a series of charts showing the reported weight loss for both procedures. Figure 3.4 shows the data. As can be seen, weight loss after a gastric bypass procedure is better than for those with the LAP-BAND™ during the first 2 years. However, by the third year the differences are small and after that there are no differences to 8 years.[20]

Although stomach stapling is an acceptable option for some people, it has proved to be unacceptable to the vast majority of those in the community who are obese, either because of its risks and invasiveness or because of the difficulties in retaining the correct settings over a long period. It can be estimated that only one of every 200 people who have severe obesity in the United States would agree to a gastric bypass or other form of stomach stapling. The other 199 either have accepted their problem of obesity or are looking for a more acceptable alternative.

FIGURE 3.4 COMPARISON OF REPORTED WEIGHT LOSS FOR ROUX-
EN-Y GASTRIC BYPASS (RYGB) AND LAPAROSCOPIC ADJUSTABLE
GASTRIC BANDING (LAGB)

The LAP-BAND™ procedure has been developed
to retain the good things that we have learned from
stomach stapling, but to overcome the problems that
made stomach stapling generally unacceptable. The
key features of the LAP-BAND™ that have led to
its acceptance are its safety, minimal invasiveness,
adjustability, reversibility and overall effectiveness.
In our practice, we used gastric bypass for many
years prior to the LAP-BAND™ becoming available,
but since 1993 we have no longer offered this option
for the first treatment of obesity as it is clearly more
dangerous, it is not adjustable or reversible and it is
no more effective in the medium term than the LAP-
BAND™. We should always seek the simple and safe

before the complex and risky. We don't crack a nut with a sledgehammer if a nutcracker is available.

In Chapter 4, we will look at all the good features of the LAP-BAND™ and discuss what are reasonable expectations with regard to weight loss. We will also look at its problems and unfavorable features. We will then describe the type of people who would be best treated with the LAP-BAND™. From this you will be able to determine whether this may be a suitable procedure for you.

CHAPTER FOUR

THE LAP-BAND™: IS IT THE BEST OPTION FOR YOU?

1. The **LAP-BAND™** works primarily by inducing a sense of satiety.

2. Its best features are the adjustability, truly minimally invasive placement and reversibility.

3. The **LAP-BAND™** treatment of obesity is a lifetime process, not just a procedure.

4. It is extremely safe but does carry some risks and a significant "maintenance" requirement.

5. The **LAP-BAND™** is the best option for obese people who have failed non-surgical treatments.

FOUR PRINCIPAL FEATURES

Four principal features of the LAP-BAND™ overcome the dilemmas that are present with procedures such as gastric bypass and other methods of stomach stapling. These are outlined below.

1. THE LAP-BAND™ INDUCES SATIETY

The LAP-BAND™ works primarily by providing a feeling of satiety, a feeling that you are not hungry. Even if you have not been eating for a prolonged period you do not feel hungry. You will wake up in the morning not feeling hungry. Food is no longer as central to your life as it once was.

When you do eat, you will get a sense of fullness after a small amount of food and so will not feel the need or wish to eat much at each meal. You will not feel as hungry between meals. The net result is that you will be happy to eat just three or less small meals per day with no eating between meals.

2. THE LAP-BAND™ IS ADJUSTABLE

This is perhaps the most attractive aspect of the LAP-BAND™. The sense of satiety is induced by the band pressing onto the surface of the stomach. By adding or removing fluid from the band we can increase or decrease this sense of satiety. At operation we place the band without any additional fluid. The tightness of the band and therefore the level of satiety is achieved by injecting some fluid through the skin into the access port tucked away under the fat of the abdominal wall.

This adjustability gives us control. Months or years after the procedure we are still able to modify the degree of satiety and restriction so that we can gently find the level that enables us to achieve the weight loss we want without creating too many unpleasant symptoms.

3. THE LAP-BAND™ IS TRULY MINIMALLY INVASIVE

LAP-BAND™ placement is a much less invasive procedure than all other forms of gastric weight-loss surgery. The band can almost always be placed laparoscopically (keyhole surgery) by passing some tubes through the skin and doing the operation through those tubes. This avoids any large incision, it avoids a lot of the handling of the gut inside and it avoids much of the pain that goes with an open operation. It enables you to get back to your normal activities more rapidly than would occur with other procedures. Furthermore, there is very little trauma to the tissues inside the tummy when placing the band. There is none of the cutting of organs and stapling things together that is needed for the other surgical procedures for weight loss.

4. THE LAP-BAND™ IS REVERSIBLE

We have no intention of reversing the procedure. If we did reverse it and took no other steps, your weight would rise. However, there are situations where you may wish to have it reversed and it is nice to know that this can be achieved relatively easily. If the band is placed laparoscopically it can be removed laparoscopically and, as nothing permanent has been done to the stomach, it will return to its normal shape.

If, therefore, in 20 years time a new magical cure for obesity is invented that is much simpler, then the band could be removed and the new treatment applied.

THE ANATOMY OF THE LAP-BAND™

Figure 4.1 is a picture of the LAP-BAND™. It consists of a silicone ring, which is placed around the very top of the stomach. The ring has an inner balloon, which is connected by the tubing to join to the access port.

The access port is placed deep under the skin on the left-hand side of the abdomen. We can feel this reservoir when you lie down and we can then put a needle through the skin into it and add fluid or take fluid away to make the ring tighter or less tight. This is the method for adjusting the degree of satiety and restriction.

FIGURE 4.1 THE LAP-BAND™, SHOWING THE SILICONE RING CONNECTED BY TUBING TO THE ACCESS PORT

Figure 4.2 shows a close-up of the ring of silicone. The inner balloon is not inflated at all and is only just visible. Notice also the locking device. This will not come undone and so the problems that occurred in the past with gastric stapling procedures, whereby the staples cut through and the effect was lost, are not expected to occur with this procedure.

In Figure 4.3, some fluid has been added to the inner balloon and you can see how the space has been reduced. This will narrow the opening from the upper

FIGURE 4.2 THE SILICONE RING OF THE LAP-BAND™ PRIOR TO THE INNER BALLOON BEING INFLATED

FIGURE 4.3 THE LAP-BAND™ WITH THE INNER BALLOON PARTIALLY INFLATED

stomach into the rest of the stomach, giving more satiety and making it more difficult to eat too much. By adjusting the amount of fluid in the balloon we can set the limits on your appetite and help you set limits on the volume of food intake.

THE LAP-BAND™ IS A PROCESS, NOT JUST A PROCEDURE

The excellent results that we have been able to achieve with the LAP-BAND™ are a team effort.

It is most important that we all see the use of the LAP-BAND™ in weight loss not just as an operation but as a process of care by a team, which commences before the band is placed and continues permanently thereafter. The surgeon, who is the leader of the team, and you as the patient, are the two key participants.

There must be a partnership between you and your surgeon. Success will only occur if both partners contribute. The surgeon must fulfill his or her responsibilities and you must fulfill your responsibilities. The surgeon must place the band accurately, and securely and safely. The surgeon must also ensure that you are able to access a comprehensive and expert follow-up process and must be sure you fully understand your role in the partnership. You, in turn, must be committed to following the rules regarding eating, exercise and activity, and you must always keep in contact with the medical team.

You should not consider having the LAP-BAND™ procedure unless you are totally committed to fulfilling your part of the partnership.

The rules regarding eating and exercise are discussed in more detail in Chapters 6 and 7. The essence of these rules is that you must have a maximum of only three small, good quality meals each day with no snacks in between. Each meal has to be solid food. The procedure does not work for liquid calories, so all liquids taken have to be of insignificant calorie content, such as water, mineral water, tea, coffee and low-calorie soft drinks. You must eat foods that have good protein content, such as meats, egg dishes, dairy products, beans and lentils, and foods that have high fiber content, such as breakfast cereals, vegetables and fruit. You must limit foods that are high in fats and especially avoid foods that contain simple sugars. Most importantly, you must learn to eat slowly and to eat a very small volume of food at each meal.

You must not only decrease your food intake but you must also increase your energy output. There must be an increase in activity and an exercise program should be undertaken on a regular basis as well as always seeking to be active rather than inactive throughout the day.

The primary focus of the LAP-BAND™ effect is on the amount of weight that is lost. We expect that, on average, people who have the procedure will lose between one-half and two-thirds of their excess weight. For example, if your current weight is 250 lb (115 kg) and your ideal weight is 130 lb (60 kg), then you have a total of 120 lb (54 kg) of excess weight. One-half of this is 60 lb (27 kg) and two-thirds is 80 lb (36 kg). Therefore, typically your weight would come down to somewhere between 170 and 190 lb (78 and 87 kg).

This is the average. Some people will have more weight loss than this and some will have less, but on average this is what we expect. We want this weight loss to occur slowly and gently. We are quite happy for you to achieve the loss of two-thirds of excess weight by 1 to 2 years after the procedure. Because we have control of the degree of gastric restriction, we have the confidence that even in later years we can still achieve further weight loss. Our aim is, therefore, to achieve the weight loss without interfering unnecessarily with the quality of life. We don't want vomiting and we don't want too severe a restriction on the normal living pattern.

The loss of up to two-thirds of excess weight is our first target. We find that if this amount of weight is lost, most of the problems associated with obesity have been solved. We can have you go on to lose a greater amount of weight if there is a good reason. For example, if you have type 2 diabetes, the more weight you lose, the less likely that your diabetes will come back. We would therefore seek as low a weight for you as possible. It is important to realize, however, that we are not aiming primarily to achieve some ideal weight. We are aiming to solve the problems that the obesity causes.

Thus, we find that in association with this weight loss many people have major improvements in their medical problems. Diseases such as diabetes, asthma, high blood pressure, back pain and other joint pains, and heartburn are greatly improved in association with the weight loss. We have measured all of these effects in many of our patients and the outcomes are summarized in Chapter 2.

Also, people become much more physically active and more flexible. They are more confident and outgoing socially. Employment prospects are improved, not only because of the improved physical appearance, but also because of the much improved capacity for physical activity and the improved self-esteem and self-confidence. The high level of self-hate gradually dissipates.

These multiple health, physical and psychosocial effects change your life. From feeling trapped within an obese body with its various problems, you quickly realize that this procedure really does work. It works without hurting you and it works over a prolonged period of time. You achieve the feeling of confidence that the problem is controlled, and that you can live a life without the illnesses and the limitations you had.

NOW WHAT ABOUT THE BAD NEWS!

It can't all be good news. There must be dangers, there must be problems, there must be failures. What are the bad things that can happen?

There are negative aspects to operations for obesity in general and to LAP-BAND™ placement in particular, and it is essential that you are aware of these.

DEATH

Any stomach operation for obesity is major surgery and carries with it the risks that would go with any complex operation. People have died from having operations for morbid obesity—it happens rarely with LAP-BAND™ placement but we can never take away the risk completely. If you are older and if you already have certain diseases due to your obesity, or if you are otherwise unwell, you will be at greater risk.

Deaths associated with obesity surgery occur mostly because of heart attacks after the operation, clots passing to the lungs or infection due to the breakdown of some part of the stomach wall. The LAP-BAND™ has been shown to be very much safer than the stapling operations, but still death might occur. If we look at the figures for LAP-BAND™ placement across the world there has been about one death for every 2,000–3,000 people who have the procedure. This is less than one-tenth of the risk of death associated with gastric bypass[21] or biliopancreatic diversion. For a death to occur, multiple things have to go wrong and go wrong in a particular sequence.

Firstly, it is extremely unlikely that anyone would die while under anesthesia. Our patients probably worry about this possibility the most and yet it almost never happens. Today, the knowledge base of anesthesia, the training and quality of our anesthetists and the presence of sophisticated monitoring systems make having an anesthetic very much safer than 50 or even 10 years ago.

If someone does die after a surgical procedure it is usual to find that a series of problems have occurred. Some injury or significant event has occurred which may not be recognized at the time. Then it is not recognized that the person is becoming unwell, the possible causes are not considered, the appropriate investigations are not done and the correct treatment is not provided. There is not just one unfavorable event but a whole series that all line up into a path.

You can minimize this risk by ensuring your surgeon and his or her supporting team are well trained, have extensive experience, can make available to you their outcome data and can show a track record of being safe. The placement of the LAP-BAND is very safe when done properly by an experienced team but its potential risks are real if they are not so well trained or proficient.

Some surgeons both in Australia and in the United States have reported that they have not been able to achieve good results. These reports are all on small series at the bottom of the surgeons' learning curves. The poor results reflect a lack of good laparoscopic skills, lack of good training in the procedure or lack of good follow-up of their patients. You should go to a surgeon who has been able to achieve good results and is proud of the outcomes. Be wary of those who try to talk you into a gastric bypass. They will try to tell you that the band doesn't work and that it causes all sorts of problems. Generally, it means that they are not confident in performing the procedure competently or that they do not want to provide the follow-up care that is so important with the LAP-BAND™.

Do not be afraid to ask your surgeon about his or her experience and outcomes. How many patients has he/she treated? Have any died? What complications have occurred? What weight loss has been achieved? How many patients have been lost to follow-up? It is your life being put at risk.

Through the Surgical Centers of the American Institute of Gastric Banding in Dallas there have been more than 7,000 LAP-BAND™ procedures performed. At the Centre for Bariatric Surgery in Melbourne there have been more than 3,500 LAP-BAND™ procedures performed. None of the people treated by either group has died. We cannot promise that a death will not occur. Often we are treating very big and very sick people. Nevertheless, the fact remains that over 10,000 people have been treated and no one has died. We intend to keep it that way.

COMPLICATIONS

There is about one chance in 50 that some compli-
cation may occur at or around the time of the operation.
Most complications are of minor significance and
do not slow your recovery. Others may be of major
significance and can be associated with a much longer
hospital stay and a much longer recovery period.
The sort of problems that are relatively common are
infections that may occur in the lung, in the stomach
in the area of the band, or at the sites where the ports
are placed through the skin.

Clots can form in the legs and some of these can pass
to the lungs, giving rise to the potentially dangerous
situation of pulmonary embolism. The stomach can
be damaged as the band is placed and perforation of
the stomach can follow. Pre-existing illnesses such as
diabetes and asthma may become more difficult to
manage around the time of the operation. We take a
range of measures to reduce the likelihood of problems
occurring but, in spite of our best efforts, we are unable
to promise that we can prevent them completely.

After the operation there is a period where a new eating
pattern must be established and during this learning
phase you may have episodes of vomiting. Ideally,
there should never be vomiting after band placement.
The force of vomiting can cause the stomach to shift

its position within the band and the effectiveness may be lost. We make special efforts to give instructions regarding eating and drinking to avoid vomiting but this ideal cannot always be achieved.

LONG-TERM PROBLEMS

As with any complex system, there is a "maintenance" requirement with the band and, on our current figures, between 5% and 10% of patients will have some-thing move or change or shift or break and will need to have this fixed by further surgery. Everything that can go wrong can be repaired, almost always by a laparo-scopic approach. Three problems in particular that we should mention are prolapse, erosions and tubing/port problems.

PROLAPSE OR SLIPPAGE

The most common long-term problem that we have had after the LAP-BAND™ procedure is enlargement of the stomach above the band. This may occur because there has been slipping of the wall of the stomach through the band (prolapse or slippage) or because of stretching of the very small stomach (symmetrical enlargement).

At operation we place the band in a very particular position and we take special measures to fix it in that position. We also strongly encourage you to eat slowly and to take a small amount of food at each meal. Every time you eat you are going to create some stretching of the small stomach above the band. If you eat too quickly or you eat too big a meal you will create a much greater stretching. If, at the same time, there is an area of the stomach wall that has not been fixed adequately, that area can slip up through the band and create a pouch above the band. We call this prolapse or slippage. If all the stomach wall is well secured but you keep eating too fast or too much, over the months and years the small stomach will stretch and remain stretched. We call this symmetrical enlargement.

If a prolapse or symmetrical enlargement occurs you will get heartburn and reflux of food and fluids. This is usually most noticeable at night. When you lie down the fluid and food that is sitting in the enlarged stomach above the band flows back up to the back of the throat. It is an unpleasant experience and can be associated with coughing and choking spells as some of the fluid trickles into the airway. If the enlargement of the stomach continues, it can eventually block off and vomiting would occur.

If it happens and will not settle with removing some fluid from the band, it needs to be fixed. This can be done but does require a further laparoscopic operation as a day patient or an overnight stay in hospital.

You are then back on track and can continue with the weight loss program.

When we compare the weight loss of those who have had a prolapse with our overall group of patients, there is no difference in the long-term weight loss. It is like you were traveling down the highway making good progress. You were diverted onto a rough track for a period and, with the revisional operation, we put you back onto the highway again. It has been very unusual for anyone to have a second slip.

The most important action you can take to avoid this problem altogether is to eat slowly and eat small amounts at each meal.

EROSIONS

It is also possible for the band to work its way through the wall of the stomach until it lies within the stomach. This is known as erosion of the band and is now quite rare. If it does occur the band ceases to be effective as it is no longer around the stomach and you will probably notice that you are able to eat a greater amount without that sense of restriction. It usually does not lead to any pain or acute illness. If an erosion happens we remove the band and repair the defect in the stomach. This may require an overnight stay in hospital. We may place a new band on a later occasion, usually after 3 months or more. This can all be done laparoscopically. Erosion has occurred in only one of the last 800 people that we have treated and so is now a rare but manageable problem.

TUBING/PORT PROBLEMS

The tubing passing to the access port can break or be punctured by the needle when we are adding fluid to the system. We use a special type of needle to make adjustments and, if the wrong type of needle is used, the access port can develop a leak. If any of these problems arise, the access port needs to be changed. This is a minor surgical day-patient procedure but does require an admission to hospital and a general anesthetic. These problems are now quite unlikely to occur because of improvements in design and technique.

CLOSING COMMENT

The risk of death is very remote, the risk of complications at the time of LAP-BAND™ placement is minor and the late problems are becoming quite unusual. Nevertheless, it is most important that you see the decision to go ahead with the LAP-BAND™ as a serious one which can only be justified if the problems associated with your obesity clearly exceed the problems that may be associated with the operation. You need to recognize your responsibilities to follow the rules and guidelines closely to minimize some of the risk of these events occurring.

FAILURE

Every medical treatment has a failure rate. Nothing is perfect and so if people claim that they succeed with every patient, whatever the treatment is, either they are not following their patients very well or they are dishonest. We define failure after LAP-BAND™ placement by three measures—inadequate weight loss, removal of the band and loss to follow-up. We measure our failure rate regularly. It is generally about 10% using these measures. Let's discuss each of these measures in turn.

INADEQUATE WEIGHT LOSS

If we have not achieved 25% loss of the excess weight by 2 years we regard that performance as inadequate and therefore a failure. On a number of occasions the patients are reasonably happy with their outcome. They may have lost 20% of their excess weight, their health is better and they are feeling improved. Nevertheless, we have to draw a line and we place it there. About 3% of our patients have failed by this criterion.

We do not give up on these people. On the contrary, we are always seeking to achieve the best possible result for all our patients, and especially for these ones.

We enter them into our "intensive care" program. We reassess them, their band, and their knowledge and compliance with the eating and exercise rules. We seek to diagnose what is wrong and then we seek to correct it. This may be inadequate follow-up or adjustments. It may be that they are eating wrongly or drinking multiple cans of soft drink, or not exercising. It may be that there is a leak in the system or there has been a slip of the stomach through the band. We identify the cause and then provide a period of intensive follow-up to get them back on track. Nevertheless, at any one time, about a third of our patients in the "failure" group are those who have not lost more than 25% of excess weight.

It is important to realize that we do not give up on you because you have not lost enough weight and that those whose weight loss is less than we would like are commenced on our "intensive care" program.

REMOVAL OF THE LAP-BAND™
We have removed the band in just over 3% of our patients. In the early days of our experience we sometimes removed the band for prolapse or erosion. This would not happen now. We have the occasional patient who asks for the band to be removed because they do not feel it is helping them enough or they do

not like the effect that it is having in some way. We discuss the decision with them carefully and if they are clear that they want it removed and they understand that their weight is likely to return to its initial levels, we will take it out. It is easy to do and if, years later, they wanted it back in again, we would be happy to at least discuss that option. There is nothing irreversible about the placement or the removal.

LOSS TO FOLLOW-UP

We are very keen that no one should be lost to follow-up. Good follow-up is one of the key elements for success with the LAP-BAND™. When we eventually track down some of those who have been lost to follow-up we note that they are frequently associated with a poor outcome. As we cannot be sure, we count these people in our failure group. At most times we are able to track between 96% and 97% of our patients, leaving 3–4% who are in the failure category because of loss to follow-up.

We work hard to minimize any loss to follow-up by stressing to you the key role that follow-up plays in the LAP-BAND™ process. We are totally committed to maintaining follow-up with you permanently. This will mean a visit at least once every 6 months.

We request a maximum time between visits of 6 months for a specific reason. A very small but definite loss of fluid occurs from the band. If you had 3.0 mL of fluid initially and we saw you again at 6 months, it is likely there would be about 2.7 mL present. You would need a small addition of fluid to get back to the correct level. Even with a loss of just 0.3 mL of fluid, you are likely to feel more hungry and to find that you can eat too easily. Weight loss will stop and you may start putting on weight. If you don't realize that this small loss of fluid is occurring, you could feel that it is your fault that the procedure is not working and be hesitant to come back because you see yourself as a "failure." This is the wrong way to think. You must come back so that we can help—by adjusting, advising, educating and sharing information.

There is a greater risk of loss to follow-up if you move interstate or overseas. If you do, please contact your surgeon with your new address and please provide your surgeon with brief information on your progress as an absolute minimum. Almost always, they will be able to introduce you to a physician in your new country or region who can continue with your care. The LAP-BAND™ procedure is not just an operation; it is a partnership with the medical team in a lifetime process. You should only decide to proceed with the procedure if you are prepared to make a commitment to this partnership and you must maintain this partnership by being in contact with us or our colleagues permanently.

There is an additional advantage in maintaining contact with us. It could be that reasons will develop in the future, either for you as an individual or for all people who have the band, which make it appropriate for some action to be taken. For example, we could find out something about the band that is so concerning that we recommend it to be removed. The LAP-BAND™ is made of silicone and there are no known side effects of having this material within the body. We have now had over 12 years of experience with the LAP-BAND™ and its placement. There have been no long-term harmful effects as long as the position is correct and you are following the rules. We will continue to monitor each person and the information about the procedure itself and, as long as we maintain contact with you, we can always advise you of any new developments.

WHO IS CONSIDERED SUITABLE FOR THE LAP-BAND™?

We take four factors into account when determining whether this might be an appropriate procedure for you. These are the current level of your weight, the problems that this state of obesity generates, the confirmation that you have made significant effort at weight loss by other means and the confidence we have that you understand what you are getting your-self into and have the commitment to fulfill your part of the partnership.

We discuss these factors in more detail below.

1. THERE IS OBESITY

Obesity is a disease that exists in our community when the body mass index (BMI) is greater than 30. A BMI of 30–35 is described as mild-to-moderate obesity. A BMI greater than 35 is described as severe obesity. Until recently, we would not wish to proceed with this procedure if the BMI were less than 35. At a BMI of 35 or greater there is a clear risk to a long healthy life, there are generally significant problems associated with obesity and there is known to be a poor outcome from any alternative therapy.

Recently, we have completed a major study of people with a BMI of between 30 and 35 and have found that those who had the LAP-BAND™ had much better weight loss, improvement in health and improvement in quality of life than a matched group who had the best program of non-surgical treatment that we could offer.[22] We are, therefore, now prepared to accept people into the program with mild-to-moderate obesity, particularly if there are medical problems associated with the obesity or if it is clear that serious and multiple attempts to lose weight have been made by non-surgical means before seeking the LAP-BAND™.

2. THE OBESITY IS ASSOCIATED WITH PROBLEMS

If there is not a problem then we don't need to look for a solution. Even if you are truly morbidly obese by our definitions, we would not wish to proceed with any treatment unless you perceived a significant problem with your obesity. This might include the physical limitations, social isolation and the medical diseases that go along with morbid obesity. It may be a fear of the effects of your obesity on your future health and life expectancy. It must be the solution that you are seeking in answer to your problems. It is not something for us to encourage just because we perceive that you have a problem.

3. THERE HAVE BEEN SERIOUS EFFORTS TRYING TO LOSE WEIGHT

It is important that you have made significant effort to reduce your weight over a prolonged period of time. The effort is likely to include supervised diets and exercise programs and we find that almost all of our patients have spent considerable time and money with the commercial weight-loss groups in an attempt to lose weight. Most have tried some or all of the weight loss pills that are available and many have been to some of the various health professionals who offer "solutions" to obesity. This includes dieticians, naturopaths, hypnotherapists, acupuncturists and psychologists.

We do not make this stipulation because we believe that these alternative lines of therapy are effective. In fact, they are almost always ineffective in the long term. We make the requirement because it is an expression of your commitment to lose weight and without that commitment we cannot be confident that you will follow your part of the partnership.

4. YOU UNDERSTAND THE RISKS AND RESPONSIBILITIES

Your weight status, the problems associated with your weight and your efforts to reduce your weight in the past are the main measures that we make. However, in addition, we will only proceed if we believe that you understand how your obesity is a problem for you, what the procedure consists of and what are realistic expectations of what it can do and what are the risks, and that we feel you are able to fulfill your part of the partnership.

The whole process of the placement of the LAP-BAND™ and the follow-up process after the procedure is a partnership between yourself and us. We are committed to do all that is necessary to get the best possible result for you and you must be committed and able to fulfill your part of the partnership. For this we need to be sure that you have a realistic understanding of the potential benefits and risks, and of your responsibilities with regard to eating pattern and exercise.

FULFILLING THE PARTNERSHIP

The surgeon has three aspects to commit to in order to fulfill half of the partnership and the patient has three aspects to commit to in order to fulfill the other half of the partnership.

SURGEON'S THREE COMMITMENTS

1. To place the band correctly and safely.
2. To ensure the patient is able to access good follow-up.
3. To teach the patient the rules to follow to fulfill their role.

PATIENT'S THREE COMMITMENTS

1. To follow the rules regarding eating and drinking, as discussed in Chapter 6.
2. To follow the rules regarding exercise and activity, as discussed in Chapter 7.
3. To come back for follow-up permanently with visits at least once every 6 months.

DECISION-MAKING TIME

Here and in Chapters 1–3 we have given you a wealth of information. We have explained how obesity is a common problem that causes many other problems to your health, quality of life and survival. We have explained the benefits of weight loss with the improvement in health and happiness and the likelihood of increased survival. Most of this information is derived from published studies of our own patients.

We have explained the different options available to treat the problem of obesity, their strengths and their weaknesses. In particular, we have given you much information on the LAP-BAND™.

We have given you a list of criteria that you could apply to decide which of these options is the best for your problem. It is now time to apply those criteria to the different options we have discussed and to see if the LAP-BAND™ stands out as the best mix of effectiveness, safety and acceptability for you.

Table 4.1 summarizes the outcomes from each of the major options for weight reduction for each of the criteria. The more pluses there are, the more that criterion is met. The perfect procedure would have three pluses for each criterion. The worst procedure would have a minus for each criterion. You will quickly see why the LAP-BAND™ is the preferred option.

TABLE 4.1 OUTCOMES FOR THE MAJOR OPTIONS OF WEIGHT REDUCTION

Attribute	Lifestyle	VLCD	Drugs	BIB™	LAGB	RYGB	BPD
Safety	+++	+++	+++	+++	+++	+	+
Effective	−	+	+	+	++	++	+++
Durability	−	−	−	−	+++	++	+++
Minimal side effects	+++	++	++	+	++	+	+
Adjustable	++	−	+	−	+++	−	−
Reversible	n/a	n/a	n/a	+++	+++	+	+
Low revision rate	n/a	n/a	n/a	++	++	++	++
Minimally invasive	n/a	n/a	n/a	+++	+++	++	+

The more pluses the better for that feature.
VLCD = very-low-calorie diet; BIB™ = Bioenterics Intragastric Balloon™; LAGB = laparoscopic adjustable gastric banding, such as the LAP-BAND™; RYGB = Roux-en-Y gastric bypass; BPD = biliopancreatic diversion; n/a = not applicable.

Table 4.1 highlights the key advantages of the LAP-BAND™ over other options—it is highly effective and yet safe; it is adjustable and reversible.

On the basis of this type of analysis, our extensive clinical experience with the LAP-BAND™ and, before that, with the gastric bypass, our awareness of the excellent outcomes that our patients have been able to achieve by using the band and the results of our numerous research studies, which have carefully and fully documented these benefits, we recommend the LAP-BAND™ as the best weight loss procedure for those who have problems arising from their obesity, who have tried non-surgical options, who understand the rules and who are committed to do their part of the partnership.

PATIENT ANECDOTE BROOKE LINDSEY

I am 26 years old and I am a registered nurse. I have lost 152 lb (69 kg) since my LAP-BAND™ surgery. I have not had plastic surgery before or since my weight loss surgery. I opted for weight loss surgery after trying a number of other methods. I tried several commercial weight-loss programs, exercise, counting calories and fat grams, and memberships at gyms. I had success with the other methods, but none of them worked long term. I was tired of living life at 292 lb (133 kg).

I had a son whom I did not want to embarrass one day. I wanted to be around to enjoy him growing up, to see him graduate and get married. I wanted to be healthy; however, the cosmetic change was a wonderful side effect. I wanted the woman on the outside to match the one on the inside. I chose the LAP-BAND™ because it was so safe. You can bet as a nurse I researched as much as I could. I loved the fact it was adjustable. If I was sick or wanted to have another child it could be adjusted and I could get the extra nutrition that I needed. I liked the idea of a slower weight loss also. I had heard with every diet I had ever been on that slower is safer.

LAP-BAND™ PLACEMENT: BEFORE, DURING AND AFTER THE PROCEDURE

1. Before placement of the LAP-BAND™ we will do a careful evaluation of your health.

2. The procedure is almost always done laparoscopically and takes about 1 hour.

3. You should be out of bed, walking around and drinking water easily at 1 hour after the procedure.

4. You take liquids only for the first week, soft foods for the second and third weeks and then solid foods after that.

5. You will return for the first adjustment of the band at about the end of the fourth week.

BEFORE THE OPERATION

After we jointly make the decision to go ahead with the procedure we will arrange for you to have some preliminary tests that are needed to document your general state of health. We may also do some specific measures of your current health problems and we will do some further tests that will minimize any risk associated with anesthesia. You will generally come into hospital either the afternoon before the procedure or on the morning of the procedure. The operation is performed under a general anesthetic and takes about 1 hour.

THE OPERATIVE PROCEDURE

The operation is almost always done laparoscopically. That means that we do not make any large incision. We pass fine tubes through the skin into the abdominal cavity. Mostly these are 0.2 in (5 mm) across, about as wide as a pencil. A special telescope is placed through one of these tubes. It has a camera attached to it so that we can see the inside of the abdomen by looking at a video screen. We pass surgical instruments through the other tubes to do the operation and we watch what we are doing on the video screen.

The band is placed around the upper part of the stomach to create a very small stomach above the band, with the rest of the stomach lying in its normal place below the band. All the food that you eat will go into this small stomach initially and then will empty slowly through the space left within the band into the rest of the stomach and onwards through the small and large bowel as normal.

An access port is placed in the abdominal wall, usually slightly to the left of center, at about the belt line. Figure 4.1 shows the access port at the end of the tubing. We can put a needle through the soft center of the access port to add saline to tighten the band. To place the access port we make a small cut in the skin, which measures 1.5 in (4 cm) in length. Therefore, at the end of the operation, you will note this small cut and also the sites where the ports passed through the skin. As the other ports are about as thick as a pencil, these incisions are quite small and, after healing, leave very little scarring.

Occasionally, the operation cannot be performed laparoscopically. This may be because the liver is too large or there has been previous surgery in the area and there are too many adhesions. Sometimes, although we start to do the procedure laparoscopically, it may be more appropriate to change to an open operation. This may occur if a significant amount of bleeding happens or if there are difficulties in passing the band around the stomach. You won't know that we have had to do this until after the completion of the operation, and you have to go into the operation recognizing that this may happen. On current experience, this will occur with less than one in 500 operations if there has been no previous surgery in the region.

If we need to do an open operation, generally you will have more discomfort after the operation and you will need to stay in hospital a day or two longer. Also, it will be a longer period before you are able to return to your normal activities. However, the procedure itself is done in essentially the same way and the end result is the same.

AFTER THE OPERATION

When you wake up from the operation you will have some discomfort. There are two main sources of this discomfort. Firstly, the sites where we passed the tubes through the abdominal wall can be sore, especially the one where the access port is placed.

Secondly, it is common to have pain at the left shoulder area after the procedure. This pain is actually coming from the diaphragm, which is the large sheet of muscle that separates the chest, with its heart and lungs, from the abdomen. It is called referred pain because, although it comes from the diaphragm, the brain interprets it as coming from the left shoulder and you feel sore there. It is common early after the operation but usually settles in a few days. Occasionally it can linger on for many weeks. We do not know exactly why it occurs and therefore we cannot predictably avoid it. Apart from letting time pass, various simple techniques have been found to help and are worth trying:

- hot packs to the shoulder
- standing or sitting upright
- resting quite still for 10 minutes
- walking about
- peppermint tea
- simple pain relievers—acetaminophen (paracetamol) or soluble acetylsalicylic acid (aspirin).

Although placement of the LAP-BAND™ is not totally painless it is not nearly as painful as if we had made a large incision. The anesthetist will have given you pain relievers before you wake up to block some of the pain and we can give you whatever additional treatment you need for pain relief at any stage. However, we will be trying to avoid too many pain relievers, especially opiate-type drugs such as morphine or meperidine (pethidine), as they can make you feel nauseous and might induce vomiting.

You will be able to start taking fluids such as water, tea or coffee as soon as you are fully awake from the anesthetic.

You will have an intravenous drip in one arm to give you additional fluids and we are happy to remove this as soon as you are drinking fluids without difficulty. Generally, we expect to remove the intravenous drip at about an hour after you come back to your bed from the operating room.

We will be encouraging you to get up out of bed and move around soon after the operation itself.

Normally, you will get out of bed and go for a brief walk within an hour of returning from the operating room.

If you do this, your recovery is likely to be smoother and easier and it is likely that you will have less problems with pain from then on. The nurses will encourage you and help you with this early mobilization initially.

Depending on where you are being treated, you may go home within 2–3 hours of the procedure or you may stay overnight. We usually do a limited barium swallow X-ray examination before you go to check that the band is in the correct position and that there is easy flow of liquid past the band. The barium swallow X-ray examination is not essential but does provide some helpful information and therefore we use it if the costs are low. In some settings it is quite expensive and then should be used only for selected patients. It involves taking just two or three mouthfuls of the barium. It does not taste great but, with the small volume, you will cope. The X-ray serves to reassure us that the band is in the correct position, shows that there is free passage of fluid past the band and provides a useful baseline record of the position of your band in case there is any problem in the future. We keep an electronic copy of this on "LapBase," our computer record of your baseline and follow-up details. It enables us to compare this X-ray with any future studies.

Before you go home we spend some time going over the rules regarding eating, particularly for the subsequent 4 weeks. We will make your initial follow-up appointments and we provide you with contact details should any questions arise once you are at home.

After you go home we would normally expect you to take 1 to 2 weeks to get back to normal activities. Even at this time, however, you may be feeling more tired by the end of the day and you will be still be trying to identify the best practices regarding eating. Nevertheless, by this time you will clearly see that you are almost fully recovered from the procedure and will already be seeing some weight reduction. You can return to work when you feel strong enough. Some will be back at work in a day or two but most will stay off work for at least a week from the procedure. We are happy for you to drive your car once you feel that you can move easily without discomfort and you can rotate enough to see about you. Normally this would be day 3 or day 4 after the operation.

EXERCISE AND ACTIVITY

We want you to start increasing activity and exercising as soon as possible. There is no physical activity or exercise you can do which will harm the band or its placement. After a laparoscopic procedure there is no weakness of the stomach muscles and so you do not need to worry about creating a problem through too much early activity. As long as your activity does not cause undue pain, please be as active as possible, as early as possible. We set no limits. We rely on your common sense.

COMMENCING DRINKING AND EATING AFTER THE LAP-BAND™

WEEK 1 AFTER OPERATION—THE "LIQUIDS ONLY" PHASE

The correct introduction of fluids and then food during the first few days and weeks after placement of the LAP-BAND™ is important in preserving the structure that we have created at operation. It is essential that we do not unduly stretch the new small stomach at this early stage, but allow it to settle in position and develop some adhesions around it, which will stabilize it for the future. It takes some time for this to occur and therefore during the first week after the operation you must take fluids only and avoid taking any solid food.

The fluid should go through quite rapidly and therefore you will probably not feel full. If, however, you do feel uncomfortably full after taking a small amount of fluid, you must not take any more until that feeling has passed. You will notice that you have very little appetite or interest in food. That is what we wish to achieve, and the less food you have, the happier we are.

At each mealtime, you should take a small amount of fluid, wait to see if it leads to any discomfort and, if not, then proceed with more. This same rule will apply later on when you are on solid food.

Notice that at this stage you will be taking calorie-containing liquids. These will be discouraged once you have moved beyond this liquid phase, but they are accepted at this stage to enable you to have some nutritional intake while at the same time not putting any stress on the system as the band settles into position. We will encourage you to continue with this pattern for at least the first week after operation.

During this time you should take no solid foods at all as this could block the pathway through the band and lead to enlargement of the stomach above the band. This is a most undesirable outcome and needs to be avoided by staying on fluids.

As you settle into a pattern of taking fluids it is most important that you become careful not to stretch the small upper stomach. This is unlikely, particularly with clear fluids, but it is something that you will always have to be conscious of avoiding. This can best be done by sipping fluids, not gulping them down.

During this first week, some people can have some nausea, headache, dizziness and lightheadedness. These symptoms are often settled with some calorie-containing liquids such as fruit juice or yogurt.

You will need to remain on fluids only for about 7 days after the operation. During this time we want the band to settle into position without any strain upon it. We therefore encourage you to avoid any solid food in case this causes obstruction at the narrow opening into the rest of the stomach, and vomiting. It is most important throughout this period that you do not generate sufficient feelings of fullness to have to vomit as this could possibly lead to movement of the band in relation to the stomach.

An ideal fluid to take through the first week is Optifast or another form of very-low-calorie diet. These are nutritionally well-balanced but low-calorie liquids without any of the sugars or fats of some other liquids you may choose. If you were taking Optifast before operation to reduce the liver size, it is a good idea to continue with Optifast through this first week, if possible.

However, some people cannot cope easily with Optifast and so alternate liquid foods need to be taken. The types of fluids that could be appropriate during this time include:

soups: avoid those with lumps of vegetable or other food within them; if you are not sure, puree the soup in a food processor
yogurt: particularly low-fat forms
milk: low-fat forms only and without added flavoring
V-8: this vegetable juice is highly nutritious
egg nogs: or other liquid forms of egg
fruits: vitamized to liquid form
fruit juices: unsweetened

pureed foods: satisfactory as long as they are liquid
fruit smoothie:
200 mL low-fat milk
100 mL low-fat yogurt
0.22 lb (100 g) fresh fruit such as banana, straw-
berry, mango
Chill all ingredients, combine in blender and blend
until smooth. Serve chilled with ice. This gives about
four serves.

- Please note that these liquid calories are not allowed
  after the early postoperative period. They are just
  for the first week only.
- Try to avoid fluids containing sugar as much as
  possible and minimize the high-fat fluids.
- Never drink sodas or soft drinks. Each can of soft
  drink has the equivalent of 10 teaspoons of sugar.
  Avoid them totally.

- Low-calorie soft drinks are allowed but let the bubbles settle before you drink or you may feel uncomfortable because of trapping of the gas.

Inevitably, with the reduced intake of food, there will be reduced bowel activity. Try not to be concerned as this is a normal expectation if the roughage is reduced. If you are truly concerned, take one of the bulk-forming laxatives such as Metamucil or Normacol, along with plenty of water. That should get things going again.

A reasonable test of the appropriateness of a fluid during this liquid phase is whether it can be sucked up through a straw. If it is too thick to do this, you probably should not be trying it yet.

If you are taking medications in tablet or capsule form during this time we suggest you try to swallow them intact initially. If there seems to be some difficulty in getting them down, you should crush them. Capsules should not be a problem as they melt at body temperature and release the medication. It is the larger tablets that are most likely to cause problems. If you do have to crush a tablet, you should check with your pharmacist first as crushing the tablet can interfere with its absorption into the body.

Drink as much water as you feel like. We do not set any particular amount to drink per day. Let your thirst tell you. If you feel thirsty, drink plenty, but if you are not thirsty, there is no need to force it. We place no maximum or minimum limits on the amount of water, mineral water, tea or coffee you drink each day.

ACCEPTING VARIATIONS IN PRACTICE

Throughout this book we describe the approach and the views that we have developed at the Centre for Bariatric Surgery in Melbourne to achieve the best outcomes for our LAP-BAND™ patients. Although our views are generally supported by all surgeons performing l AP-BAND™ placement, there will never be an exact set of rules or guidelines that are followed precisely by all. Variations may be encountered in different surgeons' practices, and this is a very healthy thing. Through variation we learn what is better and our practices can evolve. Common areas of variation include the introduction of fluids and food in the first few weeks after surgery, the use of radiological adjustments and the advice regarding carbonated drinks.

If your surgeon indicates a preference for a slightly or significantly different way of doing things, by all means discuss the variation with him or her but, in the end, you must be guided by your surgeon. No book can override the doctor–patient relationship.

This book is based on our experience, our background knowledge, our research studies and common sense. It is certain that we will not be right on all aspects but hopefully we are getting close. Our approach will evolve, as will the approach of your surgeon.

And, in spite of the variations, the skilful and caring surgeons across the world all seem to be able to achieve very similar outcomes.

WEEKS 2 AND 3 AFTER OPERATION— THE "TRANSITION" PHASE

After the first week we begin the transition from liquid foods through to solid foods. We want to do this slowly because we want to avoid any vomiting that could occur if you tried to progress more rapidly. Initially the liquid-type foods can be gently thickened up. The soups become thicker, the fruit and vegetables less pureed or vitamized, and you can start taking some of the softer foods such as eggs and the yellow vegetables. One Weetbix or equivalent might be seen as a typical breakfast. If you add a lot of skinny milk to this it is nearly liquid and is appropriate at the start of this period. By the end of the 2 weeks you should be adding less milk and it is much more like a solid meal.

FROM WEEK 3 ONWARDS—THE "SOLIDS" PHASE

After week 3 you should be on solid foods and normally you will stay on solid foods from then on. Some foods are more difficult to cope with than others. The foods that tend to be most difficult are bread, red meat and sometimes rice. White meats, particularly fish, are usually well tolerated, but initially it might be appropriate to make it with a sauce and later on delete the sauce as you move to completely solid foods. By the end of the third week you should be on solid foods and the liquids-only of the past will now remain in the past. There is one exception to this. If, due to illness or inadvertent error, you begin vomiting and have some difficulties with solid foods, it is important then to go back initially to clear liquids and come forward again through soft foods to solid foods. If this happens, you should contact the clinic and check if you need to be seen by one of the physicians.

Once you have established a diet based on solid foods you will stay with this permanently. From then on you need to avoid taking any liquids that are calorie-containing. This will then limit your liquid intake to water, mineral water, tea, coffee and low-calorie soft drinks, and maybe a daily glass of wine. Be careful initially with the carbonated drinks. The gas can build up as you cannot burp as readily after band placement as before and it can be quite uncomfortable. See how you go, letting the drink go fairly flat, and drink it if you do not have trouble. A more detailed food guide is provided in Chapter 6.

There are two final important messages:

1. If at any time during the first few weeks, or indeed at any time in the years afterwards, you feel that there is something wrong, it is essential that you get a message to your surgeon that you are worried. A number of bad things have happened to people after the LAP-BAND™ procedure because they have

consulted with someone who is not familiar with the band and who then makes a mistake of diagnosis, or treatment, or both. We do want to know if you may be in trouble. We would be very disappointed if you did not contact us and subsequently something serious happened that we might have been able to help you avoid.

2. During the first week it is usual not to feel at all hungry, to be quite uninterested in food. Please remember that feeling. That is what we want to achieve in the long term by adjusting the band. The feeling will fade away over the 4 weeks so that by week 4 you may be getting hungry, the weight loss will have stopped and the amount of food you are eating will have increased. That is normal. We then start to add saline to the system at that time and seek to move you back to the state of satiety of the first week.

EATING AND DRINKING AFTER THE LAP-BAND™

CHAPTER SIX

1. The LAP-BAND™ facilitates good eating behavior.
2. Eat slowly and eat a small volume at each meal.
3. Eat three or less meals each day.
4. Do not eat anything between meals.
5. Eat foods high in protein and fiber.
6. Do not drink any calorie-containing liquids.
7. Take a vitamin/mineral supplement.

THE KEY TO LOSING WEIGHT IS TO EAT LESS

Hundreds of books have been written by people giving you their "secret" for losing weight. In general, they talk about this type of food versus that type of food, this way of eating versus that way of eating. They are missing the point. The key to losing weight is to eat less. The volume of food is far more important than the content of the food. The body can turn almost any food into whatever it wants. Don't get lost in the detail of the type of food; focus principally on the volume of food.

We have no way of beating the laws of nature, and one of the laws of nature—the Law of Conservation of Energy—states that energy can be neither created nor destroyed. If you take in more energy (calories) than you use up, it will be made into fat, the energy store of the body. If you take in less energy than you use up, the body will use up some of its stored fat. To lose weight, you must reduce your energy intake or increase your energy output or, preferably, do both.

In Chapter 7 we will look at how you can increase your use of energy by increased exercise and activity. For now we will concentrate on the most important part of the equation—reducing your intake.

With the LAP-BAND™, you eat less. It allows you to eat less, it encourages you, it forces you, it cajoles you, it seduces you to eat less. It is like having your own personal trainer or bodyguard with you and watching over you all the time. Exactly what happens varies from person to person. For some it is easy—the fat seems to just melt away without effort. For others, it can be a struggle, with difficulties in eating correctly—eating too much or too often or too fast or making incorrect choices.

THE LAP-BAND™ WORKS BY DOING TWO THINGS

Firstly, and most importantly, the LAP-BAND™ takes away the sense of hunger and replaces it with a sense of satiety.

When the band is adjusted correctly, you will not feel hungry. You will wake up in the morning, having not eaten for more than 12 hours, and not feel hungry. You will forget mealtimes. You will not spend hours of the day thinking about food—what to have for lunch, what to buy for dinner, what you would like to have for a snack as you walk past a shop. You can get on with your day's activities without the distraction of food. We call this state of not being hungry, of having no appetite for food, as "satiety."

With this sense of satiety present most of the time, you will be happy to eat no more than three times a day. You should not eat between meals—no snacks or nibbles or just a biscuit with the coffee. If you are tempted to eat, resist it. If you cannot resist it, eat something healthy, such as a piece of fruit or a handful of nuts, and come and tell us about this.

We don't mind if you eat less than three times a day. If you do not feel like having anything for breakfast, don't have anything. Don't believe the myth that breakfast (or any other meal) is important or essential or required for good health. Breakfast is a modern phenomenon. The Stone Age person did not eat breakfast. It was not a part of the Stone Age diet. There was no food available each day until the hunter–gatherer went out and hunted and gathered.

The Stone Age man and woman could not be sure from day to day if there would be any food at all. They were programmed to cope with major variations in food intake and we all carry that same program. No significant change has occurred in this aspect of our genetic coding during the last 100,000 years. We are set up to miss meals, we are able to miss meals. So don't fight. With a little bit of help from the LAP-BAND™, you can enjoy it.

The second effect of the LAP-BAND™ comes when you do eat something. You will get a sense of fullness after a small amount of food.

You will no longer feel the need for food and can stop eating. This is called "satiation," which is different from satiety as it comes after eating. With correct adjustment of the band, the sense of satiation, of having had enough, should come after a very small volume of food, about the amount of food you could get into half a glass.

Half a glass of food! This may seem like a very small amount but it happens to be a good symbol of an ideal volume.

Half a glass of food is a realistic target. By this, we do not mean half a cup of shredded lettuce. We mean half a glass of solid food. If you are eating foods that are loose, like shredded lettuce, and therefore more space occupying, you will need to make an estimate of the compressed volume and adjust accordingly. If you are eating foods that are largely water, such as most fruit and many vegetables, you have to recognize that as you chew well and then swallow, the water will be released and passed on. The solid component of the food will traverse the area of the band more slowly.

It is important to realize that there is almost no space left above the band for the storage of food.

What you have is a "virtual" stomach rather than an actual stomach. As you eat, space for the food is created by stretching the small stomach that is there and the esophagus above it. We are wanting to avoid too much stretching or too rapid stretching. If you eat a meal too quickly or with too big a volume, you will stretch that area more than we like. If you do it repeatedly, three times a day for years, you will develop a pouch above the band which does not empty properly. Reflux of the food into the back of the throat, heartburn and vomiting can follow and we then may need to revise the position of the band. This is why we constantly stress the need to eat slowly and eat a small volume of food.

You must learn to recognize your personal satiation signals so that you know that you have had enough.

This sense of satiation is different from what you have previously experienced. Before band placement you would have had the sense of fullness more in the upper or middle part of the tummy. After band placement it is felt higher up, just below the breastbone. You must never eat to a point where this is discomfort. Stop when you are aware of it, not when it is hurting you. If you do eat too much, you may also notice some discomfort in the chest or the left shoulder. You may sneeze. You may notice that you are producing more saliva than normal and you feel a need to take a deep breath, stretch your chest up and shoulders back. Learn to detect your own particular signals of "enough" and "too much." Stop eating with the first signal and always avoid the second signal. The band has provided you with a "stop" button. Do not keep eating when it says stop.

Use this sense of satiation. Stop eating. Discard the food that Is left. No more eating until the next meal. Get on with doing something more useful than eating. Develop this as a habit. Always use a small plate. Put a small amount of food on the plate, about the amount of food that you could get into half a glass and always leave some. Never eat all the food on the plate. If you find you are wanting more, either you are eating too quickly or you need more tightening of the band.

Eat slowly.

The awareness of the sense that you have eaten enough tends to come slowly. You must learn to eat slowly so that you will sense that you have had enough before you have eaten too much. Eating slowly is one of the most important lessons that you will have to learn and one of the most important skills that you will have to acquire. Each meal should be stretched out over at least 15–20 minutes. What you haven't eaten by 20 minutes should be discarded. Make this a habit or a ritual. Always throw leftover food out. Treat this as a source of pride, not shame.

Our mothers taught us to eat everything on the plate and to stop fidgeting. Both were correct when food was in short supply, as occurred during the first half of the 20th century. You couldn't waste food as there was not enough of it. And they knew that fidgeting used up a lot of energy without serving a purpose. Wasting food and fidgeting were wasting energy when we didn't have enough. Now we have too much. Now we want you to leave food on your plate and, yes, you can fidget as much as you like—it is a great way of using up energy.

Please be reassured and reassure those around you that you will not eat too little. We have measured the nutritional status of our patients very carefully over the past 12 years and we do not find that people become malnourished. It just has not happened unless there is something seriously wrong with the position of the band. In theory it could but, in reality, it has not. There is, therefore, no lower limit to your food intake. Some nutritionists and dieticians are very focused on what, in the United States, is called the recommended daily allowance (RDA), and in Australia is called the recommended daily intake (RDI). These cover the total energy (calories/kilojoules) and the macronutrients — the proteins, fats and carbohydrates that those of us who don't have a band should eat each day. We don't have an RDA for patients with the LAP-BAND™. We do not set a minimum requirement for protein or fat or carbohydrates. However, there are minimum requirements for some of the micronutrients, such as iron, calcium and vitamins, but they can be provided without any food attached. These are discussed later in the chapter.

Our golden rule number 1 is "Have a maximum of three small meals each day." If you are eating all the food on the plate, if you are feeling that you could do with a bit more, if you looking for more food than we describe, if you are tempted to snack between meals, you must tell us. It is the signal indicating that there may be a need for some further adjustment. The key benefit of the band is the ability to take away hunger.

It will only do this if the adjustment is correct. You must call for help if you are wanting to eat too much or too often.

WHAT SHOULD YOU EAT?

What you should eat is less important than how much you should eat.

Before you start to worry about what you will eat, please never forget that the only way, ultimately, to lose weight is to eat less. The only way the band works is that it allows you to eat less. There has been so much said and written on individual foods, their benefits and their hazards — fats versus carbohydrates, saturated fats, trans-fatty acids, polyunsaturated fats, monounsaturated fats, omega-3 fatty acids, total cholesterol, "good" and "bad" cholesterol, high and low glycemic index foods, the good and bad effects of alcohol, and the need for dietary fiber. While there is good science supporting some of the claims of their health benefit or harm, there are other claims where the evidence is rather soft and there are some claims that require an act of faith as there is simply no evidence.

Let's focus on those aspects of nutrition relevant to the LAP-BAND™ and weight loss. As much as possible, this will be supported by good science but, at times, we will have to resort to common sense. We will take each of the main components of food in turn and comment on how the patient with the LAP-BAND™ should think about it.

In general, we recommend an intake that is about half of what is generally recommended by various nutritional guidelines.

We base this on extensive experience of monitoring the achievement of weight loss in several thousand patients and identifying what appears to be an optimal food intake for weight loss without signs of nutritional deficiencies. In particular, in our clinics, we regularly measure protein levels in the blood, look for changes in bone thickness, check for anemia and low iron levels, and measure vitamin B_{12} and folic acid levels. We also monitor the general health of our patients closely, particularly documenting the improvements in the diseases that their obesity had caused. From all these measures we have not been able to identify any pattern of nutritional deficiency associated with the food intake pattern that we recommend.

TOTAL ENERGY

You should take less than 1,200 calories (5,000 kJ) per day. Initially you will probably be well below this but when your eating pattern stabilizes, an intake of 1,000–1,200 calories (4,200–5,000 kJ) per day is probably about right. Because of the excess weight you are now carrying through the day, your total energy needs will be higher initially and come down as you lose weight. Eventually you achieve a balance between energy intake and energy use and your weight will stabilize at that new point.

Typically, you will lose 50–70% of your excess weight before you stabilize. You may lose 100% of your excess weight or you may lose only 30% before you stabilize. To a large extent, where you eventually stabilize will be a reflection of your total energy input. You have much more ability to vary this input than you do to vary the output. The band is there to help you reduce the input. The changes in the output (exercise and activity) are up to you.

We plan to work with you in getting your total energy input to less than 1,200 calories (5,000 kJ) per day. We can achieve this if the adjustment of the band is optimal and you follow the guidelines regarding eating.

PROTEIN

Adequate protein intake is essential. Protein provides the key amino acids that you need to maintain the body—to build tissue, replace cells, make enzymes and hormones. The fats and carbohydrates are important as the fuel to run the body. The protein provides the essential building blocks. You must get adequate protein as a first requirement. The fats and carbohydrates are the optional extras.

We estimate that patients eating optimally after placement of the band get about 30–40 g of protein per day. We have carefully monitored their protein levels. None has developed protein malnutrition and so we are happy to encourage people to continue at this level. The best sources of protein are meats, eggs, milk and cheese, beans, lentils, soybeans and their derivatives, and nuts. Red meat can be difficult for many after band placement but fish is a fine source of protein without having the high fat levels and we would prefer you to focus on fish, chicken and eggs as your main sources of protein. Minced red meat is often easy and dairy foods can also supply a useful amount of protein.

CARBOHYDRATES

Carbohydrates and fats are the fuels to run the body. They provides the energy to keep the temperature normal, to enable the organs and systems to do their work and to allow the amino acids to be made into protein. About 70% of the energy we take in is used just to keep the body working. Even if we lay perfectly still all day, we would use up that energy. The other 30% is used to provide energy for the activities of daily living. This partly explains why exercise is a relatively weak method for achieving weight loss. The exercise just affects that last 30%.

There are three forms of carbohydrates you need to consider—starches, simple sugars and roughage.

STARCHES

These are complex carbohydrates and are the main form of carbohydrates that you eat. The common foods that are rich in starches are bread, potatoes, rice, pasta and cereals. These will normally form a significant part of your food intake each day. Be careful with bread. It can tend to stick on the way down after band placement. Fresh bread, particularly, can be a problem, whereas older bread or toast may be fine. Rice and pasta can also be a problem for some. None is essential. Life will go on if you don't eat any of these foods. Use them sparingly.

SIMPLE SUGARS

These are of no particular nutritional value and add calories. It is best to avoid them. This is particularly true with the table sugar variety, known as sucrose, that goes into so many foods and drinks. One hundred years ago we ate about 1 lb (500 g) of sugar a year. Now we eat over 150 lb (70 kg) per year, 150 times more. Simple sugars fill no particular nutritional need. They are empty calories. And they are absorbed quickly as they don't need much digestion, thereby pushing the blood sugar level up rapidly. Thus, they have a high glycemic index. They are generally in a liquid form. Any soft drink is an example of a bad liquid. A 13 fl oz (375 mL) can of soft drink has the equivalent of 10 teaspoons of sugar. Other high sugar foods become liquid as soon as you eat them. Chocolate and ice cream combine the evils of simple sugars with high fat content and, being liquid, they give no sense of satiation. It would be best if you just leave simple sugars out of your diet. Unfortunately, this is not always easy as food manufacturers add sugar to all sorts of foods to increase their popularity. So you need to watch out for them. Read the food labels for total sugar content. Even a glass of freshly squeezed orange juice has the equivalent of about 7 teaspoons of simple sugar.

ROUGHAGE

Complex carbohydrates, apart from the starches, are generally not absorbed by the body and are often referred to as roughage. They pass through the gut, largely intact and make up some of the bulk of the bowel motions. It has been argued that we should have more roughage in our diets. We will not enter that debate. We are happy for you to eat high roughage foods, such as the leafy vegetables and some cereals, as long as you stay within the guideline of having the amount of food you can get into half a glass for each meal. Some people notice constipation after band placement. Please avoid or solve this problem if you are concerned by using a bulk-forming laxative, such as Metamucil, as this is a pure form of roughage without any food value.

THE GLYCEMIC INDEX (GI)

This is currently a very fashionable concept. The carbohydrates in food are broken down in the gut and absorbed as glucose. As the glucose is carried into the bloodstream, the level in the blood rises. The GI is a measure of the rate at which the food leads to increased glucose in the blood. A food is said to have a high GI if it is rated above 70, is intermediate if it is 55 to 70, and is low if it is below 55. We are still not at all sure whether the GI is of any importance for the patient with the LAP-BAND™, or for anyone for that matter. Until we know that it really matters, it is probably smart to focus on low GI foods as much as possible. Table 6.1 provides some examples of low, medium and high GI foods. More detailed listings are readily available elsewhere. Look at them but don't let them dominate your thinking. They are probably not all that important to your outcome.

FATS

Fats are our other major source of energy. They are described as "energy dense" because you get

TABLE 6.1 FOODS RATED BY GLYCEMIC INDEX (GI)

Low GI foods (<55)*	Medium GI foods (55–70)†	High GI foods (>70)‡
Skim milk	Banana	Watermelon
Plain yogurt	Pineapple	Dried dates
Soy beverage	Raisins	Instant mashed
Apple/plum/orange	New potatoes	potatoes
Sweet potato	Popcorn	Baked white potato
Oat bran bread	Split pea or green	Parsnips
Oatmeal	pea soup	Instant rice
(slow cook oats)	Brown rice	Corn Flakes™
All-Bran™	Couscous	Rice Krispies™
Converted or parboiled	Basmati rice	Cheerios™
rice	Shredded wheat	Bagel, white
Pumpernickel bread	cereal	Crackers
Pasta	Whole wheat bread	Jellybeans
Lentils/kidney/baked		French fries
beans		Ice cream
Chick peas		Digestive cookies
		Table sugar (sucrose)

* Choose these forms of carbohydrates most often.
† Have modest amounts only.
‡ Try to avoid these forms of carbohydrates.

approximately 9 calories (40 kJ) of energy from each gram of fat you eat, whereas you only get 4 calories (16 kJ) of energy from each gram of carbohydrates. Fats in the diet are made up of fatty acids linked together with glycerol. Some of these fatty acids are needed by the body because we cannot make them ourselves. You also get the fat-soluble vitamins—A, D, E and K—through eating fat. With any reasonable range of food intake you will get enough of these, so don't base your plan for food for each day of each week on this need. Try to reduce the fat intake where possible because of its energy density. Don't become obsessive about it but always prefer the low-fat options.

Fat has been getting bad press for the past 30 years as it has been taught that eating fat has led to diseases of the heart and major blood vessels. Gradually, we are achieving a higher level of understanding of which fats are bad and which are probably quite helpful. Use the following as a guide:

1. Avoid too much of the saturated fats. These are generally derived from animal sources but also coconut and palm oil. They tend to be solid at room temperature. Look for the lean or fat-free meats. Trim off the excess fat from chicken.

2. Avoid the trans-fatty acids. These occur when liquid vegetable oils are processed to become solid, and provide a good reason to minimize your use of processed foods. They are associated with a higher prevalence of heart disease.

3. In general, the unsaturated fatty acids are fine but some are better than others.

4. Among the good guys at the moment are the omega-3 fatty acids. Eating fish is the best way to get plenty of these. As fish is also our favorite source of protein, we are happy to encourage the omega-3 enthusiasm. You also get some of the omega-3 fatty acids in vegetable oils such as canola and soybean.

5. The other good guys are the monounsaturated fatty acids, as is found in olive oil. The "Mediterranean" diet has long been regarded as healthy and olive oil appears to be an important contributor. Canola oil contains these good fatty acids also.

VITAMINS

There are 13 vitamins that humans need to maintain health. Vitamins are organic chemicals that we need for normal metabolism but we are unable to make within the body. We, therefore, have to be sure that we get sufficient with our diet, and we can take a multivitamin supplement to be sure. One of the attractive features of the LAP-BAND™ is that nutritional deficiencies are not expected to occur. A good diet usually has sufficient iron, calcium and vitamins to maintain health. However, we do recommend that you take a multivitamin replacement just in case. For female patients who are menstruating or may become pregnant, this recommendation is essential. Check that the vitamin and mineral preparation has folic acid present. You should be taking at least 400 micrograms of folic acid per day. Added iron, calcium and vitamin B_{12} are also desirable.

The fat-soluble vitamins—vitamins A, D, E and K— are usually not present within normal vitamin supplements. It is important to get enough vitamin D, about 400 international units (IU) per day, as a deficiency will impair absorption of calcium and may lead to osteoporosis, a thinning of the bones, later in life. One of the best sources of vitamin D is sunlight, so a 30–60 minute walk each day provides an important extra benefit. Milk and fish are other good sources of vitamin D. We are happy for you to take up to 1 pint (500 mL) of low-fat milk per day. You can add this to your cereal, tea or coffee or just drink it. And you already know that we are keen on fish as a key part of your food intake. A small serve can provide a tasty, interesting meal of protein, omega-3 fatty acids and vitamin D.

Even with a small food intake, you should be getting enough of the vitamins A, E and K with your food. The fat-soluble vitamins are stored in the body so that taking too much can lead to harmful toxic effects.

You should not take supplements of these vitamins without medical advice.

MINERALS

Adequate daily intake of minerals is just as important as vitamins.

Sodium and potassium are taken as a part of your food and fluid intake and we have no expectation that you need any extra of these unless you have severe vomiting. Always report severe or ongoing vomiting. It is not normal after band placement. If it is happening, something is wrong. The band may be too tight, there may be a slip or prolapse, or you may be eating wrongly. It is essential that it be corrected.

Calcium is important for growth and maintenance of healthy bones. Good sources include dairy products, fish, tofu and nuts. We have measured the bone density of people who have had the LAP-BAND™ over several years and have not been able to show any suggestion of osteoporosis developing. Nevertheless, we recommend you select a vitamin/mineral supplement containing calcium as a further guarantee.

Iron can be low, especially in menstruating women. With a low intake of iron expected on a typical post-band volume of food and little red meat, we need to watch the iron levels closely and provide supplemental iron as necessary. Good follow-up and an annual blood check should be sufficient to guard against developing iron-deficiency anemia. Good food sources of iron include red meat, breakfast cereals with added iron, spinach, beans and chicken.

There is not normally a need for supplements of magnesium, phosphorus, zinc or the trace minerals.

Vitamin/mineral preparations come in different forms and you should try a range to find the one that suits you best. We would like you to take one per day but you will not comply with this if the preparation is unpleasant. Generally, the tablets are large and some people will have trouble swallowing them or getting them through the area of the band. You can find it easier to buy dissolvable, liquid and spray forms.

Berocca Performance is a good example of an ideal vitamin/mineral preparation for patients with the LAP-BAND™. It was originally made by Roche Pharmaceuticals but now is made by Bayer under the Roche label. Both are highly reputable pharmaceutical manufacturers. Berocca Performance contains all nine water-soluble vitamins in adequate amounts, has added calcium, magnesium and zinc, and comes as an effervescent tablet that dissolves to a pleasant-tasting orange drink. One a day is easy to take and covers your needs well.

FLUID INTAKE AFTER THE LAP-BAND™

Adequate fluid intake is always important. Fortunately, our thirst centers in the brain know that and tell us clearly when we need to drink. We, therefore, do not instruct you to drink a set amount of water per day. We leave it to you and your thirst center to determine the volume you need to take. Remember that there is also considerable volume of fluid in food and so our total fluid intake per day is more than what we drink. Our need for additional fluid varies quite a lot on different days. If you are having a quiet day at home in the winter you will need much less fluid than a busy outdoor day in summer. Let your sense of thirst tell you. But do listen to it and drink when thirsty.

Please try to stay with zero-calorie liquids—water, mineral water, tea or coffee (no added sugar please)— and zero-calorie soft drinks. We set no limit on how much of these you drink.

The sugar-containing soft drinks are absolutely forbidden. Fruit juices are not allowed. They are also high in sugar, low in valuable nutrients and give no feeling of fullness or satiation.

Soup is discouraged but the thicker the soup, the less unhappy we are. An occasional serve of soup is not going to be a problem. The danger with soup is that you will not get that feeling of fullness or satiation and therefore tend to take too much at each meal. However, a thick lentil or vegetable soup may well be just as effective in giving that satisfied feeling as a meal of soft foods well chewed.

Alcohol is a difficult one. Initially, we advised our patients not to take alcohol because it was a calorie-containing liquid. Also it is relatively calorie dense— 7 calories (30 kJ) per gram, which is much more than carbohydrates or proteins, which provide 4 calories (20 kJ) per gram, and closer to fat at 9 calories (40 kJ) per gram. However, many of our patients did take alcohol in spite of our guidance and so we did a study to see if they lost less weight because they were "breaking the law." To our surprise we found that, within a modest alcohol intake range, the more they had, the better the weight loss. Most were drinking wine with meals so we cannot be sure about beer or spirits. Modest alcohol intake has a number of established health benefits, such as reduction in the risk of heart disease and strokes and better control of diabetes. Since our study we have acknowledged a further benefit of a modest alcohol intake on health and have allowed up to seven standard drinks per week. As our patients were generally drinking Australian wine with the evening meal, we know a glass of fine Australian cabernet or shiraz with dinner is good for you.

PROCESSED FOODS VERSUS FRESH FOODS

Always eat fresh food if possible. Processed foods, foods that have undergone some manufacturing process, are not intrinsically bad. Some vitamins might be lost in the processing but the major food components remain intact. However, processed foods contain all sorts of additives, such as salt, sugar and trans-fatty acids. These additives do not contribute usefully to the nutritional value of the food and could be undesirable. If you use processed foods, carefully check the contents on the package. It is very useful to develop the habit of reading the labels on processed foods. Seek to understand what is in the food. Become familiar with the codes for simple sugars. Look at the amount of fats. Are trans-fatty acids present? The less the better. How much protein is present? The more the better.

CHAPTER SEVEN

EXERCISE AND ACTIVITY AFTER THE LAP-BAND™

1. An increase in exercise and general levels of activity is essential for optimal outcome with the LAP-BAND™.

2. Ensure at least 30 minutes of exercise per day but aim for 1 hour per day.

3. Walking energetically is the commonest and perhaps the best form of exercise.

4. If the back, hips or knees are wearing out, think about water aerobics, swimming or an exercise bike.

5. Be active all day. Use a pedometer to encourage you to achieve a new "personal best" often.

WHY YOU SHOULD INCREASE YOUR ACTIVITY LEVEL

Your weight loss will depend on the amount of food you eat and the amount of exercise and activity you undertake. The more you burn up, the thinner you will be.

The LAP-BAND™ works primarily by facilitating a reduced food intake. As you start to lose weight, it becomes easier to be active. The more you take advantage of that, the better weight loss you will have, the healthier you will be and the better you will feel.

The initial weight loss allows you to be more active. This activity increases the weight loss, which then allows you to be even more active. Your weight spirals down through the combination of less eating and more activity.

Conversely, if you are unable or do not increase your activity, the amount of weight loss will be less. Someone with extensive arthritis, for example, may not be able to increase activity very much and should not expect to have as good a weight loss as a result.

We will be encouraging you to become as active as possible. It is not only good for your weight loss, it also helps your health in general and it improves your feeling of well-being, confidence and self-esteem.

We suggest you think about activity in two ways—as formal planned exercise and as the activities in your normal daily living.

EXERCISE

Many of our patients have never undertaken any exercise in their life. Others have been top athletes when they were younger and have suffered the middle-aged spread. Some will have made a major achievement by spending 30 minutes a day in gentle walking. Others will become true athletes and compete in competitive sports. We want each of you to make a commitment to do the best you can. You must do something every day. Unless physically restricted by a health problem, you should seek to accumulate a total of at least 200 minutes each week in exercise.

The LAP-BAND™ does not make it easier for you to exercise but the weight loss does. With only a few pounds of weight loss you will be fitter, lighter and more able to become active.

This will make it easier for you to make the commitment—the commitment to start exercising, the commitment to continue to build your exercise program and the commitment to continue it on a daily basis permanently. We can advise and encourage you but we cannot do it for you. It is going to be up to you.

If you make this commitment and maintain a good exercise program, the benefits are extraordinary.

Weight loss is the benefit of particular interest to us in this situation but there are many others. Most importantly, exercise results in an improvement in health and you are likely to live longer. Diseases such as diabetes, hypertension and abnormal fat levels in the blood are improved sharply. Potentially fatal diseases such as heart attacks and stroke are less likely. It has been estimated that, for every mile (1.6 km) you walk, you increase your lifespan by 30 minutes. The processes of aging are slowed, with the heart continuing good function, the lungs better maintaining their ability to take up oxygen, and the bones remaining strong. The lapses of memory are fewer, sleep is improved and depression is less likely. The sense of well-being and health improves your quality of life. You will think more clearly, and work with more energy and stamina.

There are many different forms of exercise and it is worth identifying which exercises best enable you to achieve the optimal results. In general, we want you to put most effort into doing those exercises that go under the descriptors of "aerobic" or "cardio." The other forms are strength and flexibility exercises. The aerobic exercises are those that use the large muscle groups continuously for prolonged periods. Vigorous walking is perhaps the best example. Other types of aerobic exercise are bike riding, swimming and jogging. If you go to the gym, do those activities that involve low-to-moderate effort but which are repetitive, going on for several minutes. You could do a "strength" program using heavy weights and a few repetitions to gain power and body shaping. However, this is not what we are after. The central feature of the aerobic exercises is that they use most of the major muscle groups in the body, in a way that pushes up your heart rate and gets you breathing more quickly and deeply.

We want you to try to exercise each day. Make it a part of your life, plan for it, look forward to it and enjoy it. If you are doing something that you do not like, you will find excuses to miss it. Soon it is no more. Find the activities that you enjoy. Create some variety. Encourage others to exercise with you. There are few things more powerful in keeping you on your program than the commitment to meet a friend for the activity. Personal trainers are excellent in optimizing your program and providing the stimulus to keep you at it.

You should seek to do at least 200 minutes of exercise each week. Ideally, this would be achieved by doing 30 minutes on each day of the week. If your other commitments do not allow for daily exercise, you can exercise on three weekdays and make up the difference on the weekend.

It is not necessary to do the 30 minutes in one block. It is equally effective if the exercise is divided into two blocks of 15 minutes or even three blocks of 10 minutes. Surely there are few of us so busy that we cannot squeeze in three 10-minute blocks of exercise each day. Just walking up 20 flights of stairs in your office building would do it. Walking 1 mile (1.6 km) down the street would do it. Riding your exercise bike for 10 minutes would do it. Just do it.

The most common exercise and one of the best is walking. For those who haven't exercised, it is certainly the best starting point. Some of you will be limited in your ability to exercise because of health problems. Osteoarthritis involving the hips, knees or feet is a common example but there are many others. If you are disabled with arthritis, the effort for you to walk once around the house may be equal to the effort for a healthy person to walk for 30 minutes. As long as you make the effort, you use up energy and you help your weight loss. Do the best you can.

For those who are not physically limited by diseases such as osteoarthritis, we would be looking for you to do a minimum of 30 minutes of walking each day. Ideally, you will build up to 1 hour per day. If walking is your preferred activity it should be a brisk walk, enough to get your pulse rate up and your breathing going. If you are doing it with a friend, it is not a stroll and a chat. It is stepping out, and conversation should be a little difficult. Make a note of how far you go and how long you take and try to improve progressively. There is no upper limit on exercise.

All forms of exercise are allowed.

There is no exercise that is excluded because of the band. You cannot hurt or move the band by exercise. The access port is under the skin and it can be tender in that region. Getting bumped there may be uncomfortable. But you cannot hurt the port itself. It is far too robust. The band itself is totally remote from any point of contact and cannot be damaged by any physical activity. Sometimes, when you are joining a gym and you tell them you have a LAP-BAND™, the staff may be unsure of the limits placed by the band. They may even request a physician's certificate to guide them about the implications. Please reassure them. There is nothing that can happen to the band or the port. There is no need for a certificate. Just get going.

Look for variety in what you do. Keep it interesting. Do some of those activities that you have missed because of your weight problem—a hike in the local national park, a bike ride, kicking the football with the kids, swimming or surfing at your local beach, horse riding. Table 7.1 provides just a sample of the options. Try them all and add to the list. Remember that these activities are good in every way—good for the effectiveness of the band, good for your health, good for your quality of life and good fun. These include the things you missed out on because of your weight. Go for them now.

If you are limited in your activities by pain in the back, hips, knees or feet, look to the non-weight bearing exercises. Water aerobics and swimming are excellent

TABLE 7.1 THE ACTIVITIES OPTIONS

Walking, jogging, running	Riding horses
Bike riding—road bike	Rowing, canoeing, kayaking
—mountain bike	Skiing—downhill, cross-country
—exercise bike	Football—Australian Rules, Rugby, American football, soccer, hockey
Bush walking/hiking	
Aerobics—at the gym or at home	
—water aerobics	Basketball, netball, volleyball, racquetball
Stretching exercises	Baseball, softball
Dancing—any style, no style	Roller-blading, roller-skating, ice-skating
Swimming	
Tennis, squash, table tennis	Having sex—not to be underestimated
Golf (no carts please)	

activities. Riding an exercise bike might be possible if walking is difficult.

PERSONAL TRAINER

If you can afford it, a personal trainer is invaluable, especially as you get started. The personal trainer should be able to evaluate your particular abilities, needs and interests. He or she can then establish reasonable goals, design a program of exercise that is optimal for you to reach those goals, and guide you in correct technique. Most importantly, the personal trainer provides the motivation to keep you reaching your goals.

THE EXCUSES FOR NOT EXERCISING

There are many things that seem to get in the way of an exercise program. You miss your planned activities for what you feel are perfectly good reasons. We hear them all the time. After placement of the LAP-BAND™ a number of excuses are disallowed, forbidden, not recognized, not permitted. All of the following excuses are on the disallowed list:

- I had the flu.
- I just didn't have time.
- I was on holidays.
- I was overseas.
- My mother/husband/kids were sick.
- I am not thin enough yet.
- I can't afford to go to the gym.
- I have no one to look after the kids.
- I work all day every day.
- Any other excuse not listed.

None is allowed. You must exercise. It must be given priority. Picture the cartoon of the doctor asking his busy executive patient: "Which fits into your busy schedule better—exercising one hour a day or being dead 24 hours a day?"

ACTIVITIES OF DAILY LIVING

Formal exercises, such as the ones we have listed in Table 7.1, are really only a small part of the energy we use each day in being active. Most of the energy is used in the simple activities of daily living.

Activities of daily living include walking around the house, going to work or shopping, doing the things we need to do. You can increase your energy use quite a lot by increasing these activities.

Get up earlier and keep active through the day. Regard sitting down as a wasted opportunity. Be standing rather than sitting. Be walking rather than standing. Be outside rather than inside.

Look for excuses to be more active. Park the car at the back corner of the car park of the shopping center, rather than waiting for a spot near the entrance. Or better, leave the car at home and walk to the shops. Use the stairs, not the escalator. Get involved in activities in the community. Do things with the family. Take up a sport. Become a tourist in your own community by visiting and revisiting all the interesting places.

Use temperature to help. We use a lot of energy just keeping our body temperature within its normal range. In an air-conditioned environment of about 70°F (21°C), you will be using the least amount of energy for temperature control. If the temperature is higher or lower than 70°F (21°C), you will use energy to maintain your body temperature. Leave the air conditioner or heating off. Be outside as much as possible where the temperature is whatever nature has determined. You are much more likely to be active when you are outside. We tend to keep moving, doing things, when outside, whereas we tend to sit when inside.

As your weight comes down, your capacity to do things becomes much greater, partly because you have less weight to carry, partly because of improved health and partly because of the psychological feeling of relief that a problem that has been the bane of your life has disappeared. Use this increased enthusiasm for activity to do all the things that need to be done, and then look for more.

A pedometer is one way of getting feedback on how active you are. The pedometer is meant to encourage you to be active. Use it as a stimulus to show that you are improving. Make sure that today you do more than yesterday. Make sure that this week you are more active than last week. You should seek to exceed 10,000 steps per day. Always be trying to achieve a new personal best.

PATIENT ANECDOTE DAN FORD

I played sports growing up and through high school. My activities kept me in shape and my weight down. When I got out of school I got out of sports. Time, family and other priorities took over my life. Although I longed for the teamwork, camaraderie and, more importantly, the physical fitness involved with sports, my weight would not allow me to participate at the level I wanted to. I have tried all the fad diets. Some with little or no success and others with marked success until I could no longer either afford them or continue to structure my life around diets that did not allow me to participate with my family. Food is life. Almost everything we do has food associated with it. The fad diets that did work only brought more guilt when the weight came back and with it disappointment and failure, which always seemed to go hand in hand with dieting.

I then I learned about the LAP-BAND™. I had trouble at first believing that with the band the weight would not come back, that it was not a diet but a tool, and that I was in total control of my weight loss. Even better than that, once I hit my goal the band would be there to help me maintain that weight for the rest of my life. As a bonus, all the sports and family activities I had missed out on for over 20 years would be within my reach.

I had my surgery May 12, 2005. The surgery went perfectly and I actually went into work the following day to check on appointments and messages. I had no pain whatsoever. Although my results are not typical, I hit my goal within 5 months! Down 170 lb (77 kg)! A world of opportunities has reopened for me. There is nothing I can't do. More importantly, there is nothing I can't experience with my children. All the things I stayed away from I can now do. Whether it's playing softball with my daughter or ice-skating with my son, who plays ice hockey. The LAP-BAND™ has given me my life back. It had been so long I had almost forgotten.

ADJUSTING THE LAP-BAND™

1. The adjustability of the LAP-BAND™ is its most important feature. We should use it skillfully, wisely and with enthusiasm.

2. We are seeking a state of satiety, of not being hungry, of not being interested in food, of being in the "green zone." Work with us.

3. Too little fluid in the band is wasting the opportunity. Too much fluid is harming the process.

4. There will always be a need for some fine adjustment. Therefore, there is always a need for follow-up consultations.

ADJUSTABILITY OF THE LAP-BAND™

Without doubt, the best feature of the LAP-BAND™ is its adjustability. Optimal adjustment of the band is the key to effective weight loss.

You need to understand this process to get the best results.

When we place the band during the operation we usually do not add any additional fluid to it. All the free space within the band is filled with saline before we place it, but it is at zero pressure and there is no added fluid. Only occasionally, when we may feel it is too loose, will we add some additional fluid. We want you to get over the operation without having to cope with a very tight band at the same time. In particular, we hope that you do not have any difficulties with swallowing fluid or food and have no vomiting early after placement of the band. The initial 4-week period after operation is set aside for the band to settle into position and for the surrounding tissues to become firm so that there is less chance of the band moving at a later time.

THE FIRST 4 WEEKS

We generally start to add saline to the band at about 4 weeks after placement. During the first 4 weeks you are not going to be feeling very hungry and you will be losing weight. In particular, it is usual for you to feel no hunger or interest in food during the first week and most of the weight loss occurs at that time. During the next 3 weeks the feeling of hunger and interest in food returns and the weight loss slows or stops.

Remember that feeling of lack of hunger and lack of interest in food during the first week. That is the sense of satiety that we will be seeking to reproduce. We will be looking to return you to that state of satiety by adjusting the band. If you remember it well, you can guide us. You can say if you are not back to that point or alternatively you can recognize that you have returned to the same level of satiety as in that first week.

Typically, by the end of that 4-week period, you will notice that you are eating too easily, you can eat larger amounts of food than you thought you should be eating and you may be getting hungry between meals. This is normal. These are the signals that you need fluid added. We will start this at 4 weeks. The amount of fluid we add depends upon a number of factors and is really a medical decision. It will depend on the type of band you have, the amount of hunger or satiety you have experienced during the 4 weeks, the weight loss that has occurred and the approach to adjustment used. Normally, for the 9.75 cm and 10 cm LAP-BAND™, we will add between 1.0 mL and 1.5 mL. For the LAP-BAND™ VG series we will add 3.5–4.0 mL and for the LAP-BAND™ AP series we will confirm that a baseline amount of 3 mL is present and then add between 1.0 mL and 1.5 mL to give a total volume of 4.0–4.5 mL.

It is worthwhile being aware of the approximate amount of fluid in the band but please do not focus on this too much. There is nothing magical about any particular volume and there is no reason to believe that the volume your friend has is any better than what you have. The key to the adjustments is to achieve the feeling of satiety, of non-hunger, of disinterest in food. Whatever volume of fluid is needed to achieve this is the correct volume. Increasing the volume beyond this is likely to harm, not help. You will be in what we call the "red zone" (see inside back cover). Too much fluid and that is where you will be.

In the LAP-BAND™ world on the Internet, in the discussions across Web sites, there has built up a concept of "the fill" as if this is the be-all and end-all. It is not. Correct adjustment is so much more than going to a "fill center" and getting a "fill." It is a real clinical consultation. It involves sitting down with someone knowledgable and experienced, usually a physician or nurse practitioner, talking about your eating pattern, talking about any difficulties, reviewing for symptoms that something might not be quite right, looking at the weight loss, giving advice regarding eating, exercise and activity and, after all of that, maybe making an adjustment. The adjustment is a part of the clinical consultation; it is not a procedure independent of clinical assessment.

With the addition of fluid we are looking to achieve two effects—satiety or the feeling of not being hungry even when you haven't been eating, and satiation, the feeling of being satisfied after eating. The effectiveness of the band will vary depending on whether we are near to the optimal setting for the band or not. Whether you feel a sense of satiety and satiated helps us know if we need to add more fluid at each visit or whether we are close to the optimal setting. It is very important that you understand these effects. If you do, you are able to work with the band to get the best result and you can guide us in achieving a correct balance for you.

1. SATIETY

The first effect of adding fluid is that you will feel less hungry.

You acquire a feeling of satiety, which is another way of saying that you are not hungry or have no appetite for food.

This is the most important of the two effects and is the principal reason why the band works so well. For many of our patients, it will be the first time in their life when they can remember not feeling hungry. They are not thinking about food. They are not looking to eat and they can go for many hours without eating because they simply don't have any interest in food.

This feeling of satiety will enable you to stick to the rule of not having more than three meals per day. We don't mind if you have less than three meals per day but we do not want you to eat more than three times. Not even a biscuit or piece of fruit. If, after an adjustment, you find that you are still looking for a snack between meals or even feeling hungry, tell us and we can add more fluid. This is one of the important markers to us that you need more fluid.

2. SATIATION

The second effect of adjustment is to give you a feeling that you have eaten enough, after taking only a small amount of food.

This is called satiation, a sense of being satisfied by the amount of food that you have eaten.

If the amount of fluid added is optimal, you will eat only a small amount and be comfortable. We want you to stop eating at that point. Do not go on and eat until you feel full. By then you will have eaten too much. Eat just enough to take away any feeling of hunger and then stop.

To achieve satiation, you must eat slowly. The signals from the stomach to the brain to tell you that you have eaten enough pass only slowly. How often do you recall feeling like an extra serve of some nice food, eating it, and then, 20 minutes later, regretting that you ate the extra bit as you now feel too full. It takes 10 to 15 minutes for the feeling of satiation to become clear. We really don't want you ever to get that full feeling. For a start, it means you are eating too much and if you keep doing it you will stretch the new "mini" stomach, which will get larger as a consequence and then we may have a problem. And you will not be losing the weight that we want you to lose. Two bad outcomes from eating too much, from eating to fullness rather than to the point of not being hungry.

The best strategy to enable you to eat only just enough food and to recognize the sense of satiation is to always use a small plate, put a small amount of food on the plate, eat slowly and always try to leave some. Let's call this the "angel's share." Try not to eat everything on the plate. Get in the habit of throwing out food. Leave some for the angels. If you haven't left some food on the plate, you may need a further adjustment. It is especially important to eat slowly. Even though there is only a small amount of food, stretch each meal out to 15 to 20 minutes. Play around with the food. Push it around the plate. Stop after each bite and consider if you need any more. If you are no longer feeling that you need any more, stop and discard what is left. If you are still feeling you need more, take another bite and then reconsider.

Chew well, don't gulp the food down. The two worst eating practices you could have are to eat too quickly and to eat too much volume. These will stretch that new "mini" stomach and, if you keep doing it repeatedly, eventually the stomach above the band will stretch and this may need fixing surgically.

You will be amazed at how little you need to eat and how little you will feel like eating. As a community we all overeat. Almost everyone eats too much but some are fortunate to be able to burn off the excess energy and therefore not put on extra weight. However, more and more of us are storing some of the extra food as fat and that is why about two-thirds of the adult population are now either overweight or obese.

Once you have the band, those around you, especially your family, will notice how little you are eating and may worry that you should eat more. They can sabotage your best efforts through this misunderstanding. You must resist any pressures to eat more than we recommend. The pressure may come from your family, your friends, your work colleagues and even some of the health professionals that you may see. Learn to recognize what is happening and put up your guard against it.

Be polite but firm. Don't be seduced. They may have only good intentions. They may have bad intentions and, through envy or whatever reason, are truly trying to sabotage your efforts. Stick to the rules.

As described in Chapter 6, you should eat the amount of food you can get into half a glass. If you are eating or wanting to eat more than that, we need to consider adding more fluid to the band. Use the image of the amount of food you can get into half a glass as you serve yourself. Use a small plate and, if possible, a small spoon or fork. Serve yourself away from the table. Do not have the food served at the table. It is too easy and tempting to have a bit more. Take your small serve to the table, eat it slowly, push it around, play with it, take very small bites and leave some for the angels.

Think of strategies that help you eat slowly. Talk with your family. Read at least one page of a book or a newspaper article between bites. Do knitting. Watch television. Anything that helps you to eat slowly, to stretch the meal out to 15 or 20 minutes.

HOW TO GET TO KNOW AND LOVE THE "GREEN ZONE"

The "green zone" is a concept developed within our group to explain visually where we are trying to get to with our adjustments. It is well worthwhile studying the figure on the inside back cover and understanding it. You can then place yourself somewhere in or between zones. Your view of where you are helps us decide about adding or removing fluid from the band. We have put the "green zone" figure on the inside back cover so that you can find it easily. It is a key concept in the adjustment process. Please get to know it, to understand it, and to love it. Refer to it frequently and always try to estimate where you are along the scale.

Let's discuss what the figure illustrates.

1. **The yellow zone**. You are in the yellow zone if you have not had enough fluid added to the band. There is too much space within the band for food to pass through and too little effect of causing satiety and satiation. You may still get hungry and look for food between meals (lack of satiety). You may be inclined to eat too much at a meal and not leave any for the angels (lack of satiation). You may be having no weight loss or it may not be as rapid as we would like. This is common during the first few weeks after the placement of the band. Our main aim with the initial series of adjustments is to get you out of the yellow zone and into the green zone.

2. **The green zone**. This is the target zone. This is where we want you to be. In the green zone you are

not hungry. Food is not of much interest and you spend little time thinking about food, or meals or what you will have for dinner or what you will buy at the supermarket. You simply have lost interest. When you do eat, you will notice that you do not feel like eating much. You will feel comfortable and not hungry after a small amount of food. You should be able to eat a fairly broad range of food but some foods like red meat, fresh bread and rice can be difficult. You can place a small amount of food on a plate, maybe equal to the amount of food you could get into half a glass, and you will be happy to leave some. Once you have finished the meal you are not interested in eating anything until the next mealtime. Your weight should be dropping by about 2 lb (1 kg) or more per week early after the operation and about 1 lb (0.5 kg) per week after 6 months or so.

3. **The red zone**. You go into the red zone if we make the band too tight or if there is something wrong with its position which causes an obstruction. Eating solid foods becomes more difficult. You prefer softer or liquid foods. The range of food that you can eat becomes limited. Many good foods are not able to stay down. Foods will "stick" at the lower part of the esophagus. You feel a tightness at the lower chest. You may vomit or need to go to the bathroom and bring up what seems to be stuck. Soft slippery foods like chocolate and ice cream become preferred. They

can slide down, whereas the good foods cannot. We call this "maladaptive eating." It does not occur because you are evil and not cooperating and cannot follow a simple, clear set of rules. It occurs because the band is too tight. If the band is too tight, people can actually put on weight because they are eating the wrong foods. We can take out some fluid and the weight loss gets going again. This may seem curious but it is typical of what happens when people have moved into the red zone. Stay out of that area or, if you think you may have slipped into it, talk to us and we can see if removal of some fluid is needed.

Note that more fluid in the band is not necessarily better. It is common to meet patients with the LAP-BAND™ who believe that the more fluid we add to the band, the better the weight loss. You can see discussion of this in chat rooms on the Internet and you see people become concerned because they have less fluid than someone else. From this discussion of the green and red zones we hope that you can see that this is not true. Too much fluid in the band can be harmful. Finding the correct setting for you and then maintaining you at that level is the main challenge of the follow-up period. It requires clinical assessment and careful clinical judgment. The final decision of making an adjustment and of how much to add is a medical one but you are able to guide us considerably by understanding what we are trying to achieve.

THE PROCESS OF ADJUSTMENTS

People worry about the adjustments, particularly before the first one. Some of our patients have said they worried more about that first adjustment than they did about the operation. There is something about getting jabbed with a needle that just does not appeal to everyone.

Please don't worry. It is not that bad. It should be about the same as having a blood sample taken for testing. Both generally are straightforward and involve a single stab and then it's over. On occasions both can be difficult but hopefully not for you.

WHAT HAPPENS WITH AN ADJUSTMENT?

OFFICE ADJUSTMENTS

We recommend doing the adjustments in the consulting room. You lie on the examination table with a pillow placed under the middle of your back. This pushes your tummy up and makes it easier for us to feel the port. Once we feel the port, we usually put a mark on the skin directly over it using a marker pen. This indicates where the needle should be placed. We put some antiseptic on the skin and, while that is working, we select the length of needle that should be able to reach the port comfortably and attach it to a syringe that is appropriate for the fluid volume of the band at that time. We pop the needle through the skin. This is usually the only bit of pain. It should be no different from having a blood sample taken for a blood test.

The needle then passes through the fat under the skin down to the surface of the port. As fat has very few nerve fibers that detect pain, this is usually pain-free. We then get you to cross your arm across your chest and lift your head up off the bunk. This causes the muscle layer to which the port is attached to become quite firm and makes it a lot easier for the needle to go through the injection plug of the port.

Once the needle is inside the port, we draw out all of the fluid into the syringe so that we can measure the volume, making sure that it is the volume we expected, that there is none missing. We then add that fluid back in and also add the additional fluid that we have agreed is needed. We then withdraw the needle and may place a Band-Aid over the spot. Generally the procedure takes only 2 or 3 minutes.

RADIOLOGICAL ADJUSTMENTS
While we almost always do the adjustments in the office, some groups prefer to do the adjustments in the radiology department. The needle is put into the port while imaging with X-rays. You then stand in front of the X-ray machine and drink some liquid barium.

They watch this pass through the area of the band. Fluid is added to the port until there is only a narrow column of barium passing through. The needle is then removed.

We are not in favor of the radiological method as the costs are higher, it requires much more of your time and ours, and you will get quite a dose of radiation with multiple adjustments. We see the adjustment as just one part of the clinical consultation. The office model lends itself to that, whereas adjustments in radiology tend to be just a "fill" and any clinical discussions and assessments generally will have to occur elsewhere. We have no data to suggest that there is any better or worse outcome with either method. We therefore prefer to keep it simple and safe.

AFTER THE ADJUSTMENT

We make the adjustments in a stepwise fashion over many weeks, seeking slowly but progressively to get to the correct setting. It is simply not possible to go directly to the final volume. You would certainly be blocked off or at least in the red zone. After each adjustment, there is an adaptation, a settling in, a molding of the band and the stomach. After an adjustment, typically you will feel quite tight in the area for 2 or 3 days and then you will notice it gets easier.

You may have trouble taking solid foods and have to go back to soft foods or even liquids for these 2 or 3 days. We don't insist that you do that. We are happy to leave it to you to decide. If you are struggling with solid foods, go back to the softer foods. If you cannot cope with the softer foods, go back to liquids only. If you cannot cope with liquids, come back to the clinic to have some of the fluid removed. We must have added too much too quickly. On most occasions you will notice a significant difference after an adjustment but will still cope with solid food. After 2 or 3 days you will find it a little easier but hopefully still significant and you will be eating less than before the adjustment.

MAKING THE DECISION TO ADJUST

This is very much a joint decision. You will know if you are still hungry, if you are eating too easily and maybe too big a volume, and you will sense that you are not losing weight fast enough. We will be asking you about hunger, appetite, volume and type of food, and presence of symptoms such as vomiting or heartburn, which could indicate that you are in the yellow or red zones rather than the green zone. We will measure your weight and look at how much you have lost since the last visit. We will also be looking at your overall rate of weight loss.

It can happen that you do not lose much weight over a 2- or even 4-week period yet we are happy with your overall progress because you had lost more weight than expected at an earlier time and you are on track to achieving our target for weight loss. There can be fluctuations in the rate of weight loss at times for poorly defined reasons. If your overall weight loss is fine, we are not necessarily going to react to any single period of slow weight loss. We see your progress toward our targets very readily on "LapBase," our computer record of your baseline and follow-up details, and can show you whether you are on track to your target or not. This is a great help in deciding whether you need further adjustments and of reassuring you after a slow month. It also shows clearly if we are going too slowly, in which case we will review your eating and exercise patterns, and consider adding more fluid to the band.

If we both agree that you are not in the green zone, we are keen to adjust the band so that you get there as soon as possible. The actual volume of fluid that is in the band is important to us and we document it in LapBase. However, we do not want you to focus on it unduly. There is nothing magical about any particular volume. The best volume is the one that gets you right into the green zone. It depends on you and on the type of band you have. It has no relation to anyone else. The fact that your friend or someone in a chat room on the Internet has a different volume is not relevant.

Your first adjustment after the placement of the LAP-BAND™ is usually at 4 weeks for two reasons, as stated above. Firstly, 4 weeks is expected to be enough time to allow the band to settle into position. Secondly, you are usually starting to get hungry by then. During the first week after the operation you would normally find that you don't feel hungry at all. You have no interest in food and couldn't care whether you eat anything or not. We want you to recognize that feeling and remember it. That is the feeling of satiety that we will be seeking to restore with the adjustments. If you can remember what it feels like, you can tell us when you have reached that point again during the later adjustments. By the second or third weeks after operation you will be losing that feeling of satiety and the good initial weight loss will have slowed. By the fourth week, when you are usually getting hungry and are not losing any more weight, it is time to step in and start the adjustment process.

From the first adjustment at 4 weeks, visits should occur at 2-weekly intervals until you feel that you are in the green zone. This may require two to four more visits. After each adjustment you are likely to feel an exaggerated effect for the first 2–3 days before settling into a new level of satiety and restriction. By the end of the week after an adjustment you are usually able to recognize if you are sufficiently restricted. We could arrange to see you and do further adjustment at that time but usually we prefer to wait an extra week to allow you to be sure of the effects on appetite and eating and to allow us enough time to check your weight loss over a longer period.

As we get nearer to the green zone we can stretch out the interval between visits to 4 weeks, 6 weeks, 3 months and eventually to 6 months. We do not want to ever have a gap of more than 6 months between visits. Remember the eighth of our golden rules is "Always keep in contact." You must always be coming back for check-ups, with 6 months the longest duration between check-ups that we would like to happen. At all visits, doing adjustments is just one of the tasks we want to do. We also want to discuss your eating practices and your exercise program. We want to check whether you are taking supplements of vitamins and minerals. We want to inquire about symptoms that could indicate the band is too tight or misplaced, and we want to be checking on the activity of your other health problems and their treatments. Please do not see these visits as solely for "a fill." They should always be proper medical consultations and adding fluid to the band is just one of many important tasks to be completed.

Nevertheless, keeping the volume of fluid in the band is one of the most important tasks and it will remain so even years after the band has been placed. You should always expect that there will be an ongoing need for further adjustments for two reasons. Firstly, there is a continuing process of adaptation or molding of the band and the stomach. What was tight enough at one time may be too loose 6 months later. Secondly, there is a slight loss of fluid from the band over time. If you had 7.0 mL placed at an adjustment, you could expect that 6 months later that volume may have dropped to 6.7 mL. That small loss of fluid is enough to lead to overeating. If you were unaware of this small fluid loss, you may think that you are failing and blame yourself. In reality, you just need a top up. That gets you back into the green zone.

WEIGHT LOSS AFTER THE LAP-BAND™

1. Weight loss is the first, and the most important, measure of the effect of the LAP-BAND™.

2. We aim to have everyone lose two-thirds of their excess weight.

3. Weight loss should occur slowly, stretching out for 1 to 3 years after placement of the LAP-BAND™.

4. Failure to lose enough weight will occur if the adjustments are not correct or you are not following the eating and exercise rules, or the follow-up visits are not frequent enough.

QUESTIONS ABOUT WEIGHT LOSS

The primary reason for having the LAP-BAND™ placed is to lose weight. Through weight loss, there should be an improvement in your physical and mental health, you should have a better quality of life and you can expect to live longer.

Questions foremost in your mind as you anticipate the benefits of the LAP-BAND™ probably are:

- How much weight will I lose?
- How quickly will I lose it?
- Could I fail to lose enough weight?
- What must I do to get the best weight loss?

Let us discuss each of these questions in turn.

HOW MUCH WEIGHT WILL I LOSE?

On average, people will lose between 50% and 60% of their excess weight.

Our patients typically have 125 lb (57 kg) of excess weight. If you are this "typical" person, you should lose between 60 and 80 lb (27 and 36 kg) in weight.

If your starting weight is lower, that is, you have less excess weight, you will lose fewer pounds (kilograms) but probably a greater percentage of your excess weight. If you are bigger, that is, you have more excess weight, you are likely to lose more pounds (kilograms) of weight but a lower percentage of your excess weight simply because there is so much more to lose.

As an example, let us compare the outcomes for someone weighing 600 lb (272 kg), who has 450 lb (204 kg) of excess weight, with someone who is 220 lb (100 kg) and has 65 lb (29 kg) of excess weight. If the first person lost 225 lb (102 kg), they would have lost 50% of the excess weight, whereas the second person could lose just 33 lb (15 kg) and would also have lost 50% of excess weight. You could regard both outcomes as about equal and yet the numbers are quite different. When we indicate a particular weight is a realistic target, we are taking into consideration your initial weight.

It is important to understand how we calculate your excess weight and how we set the targets for weight loss. It is also important for you to realize and accept that we are not aiming to have you lose all of your excess weight. We are aiming to improve your health and your likelihood of living a full length of life, without the physical and psychosocial disabilities that obesity causes.

We regard the normal weight for the population as being a BMI of between 18.5 and 25. If you have a

BMI of 25, you are at the upper limit of normal. Any weight above that is excess to normal. We therefore calculate the weight you would have to be to have a BMI of 25 and subtract that value from your current weight. The difference is the excess weight. As you lose some of that excess weight we often describe this as a percentage, using the term "percentage of excess weight lost." For instance, if your excess weight is 130 lb (60 kg) at the time of band placement and you have lost 65 lb (30 kg), you would have lost 50% of your excess weight.

We set several targets for the amount of weight reduction we would like each person to achieve.

These targets are calculated automatically on "LapBase," the computer database that we have developed to assist us in following your progress. The first target is to have you lose two-thirds of your excess weight. We set this target when we were beginning to use the LAP-BAND™ back in the early 1990s. We now have measures on several thousand patients and we know that, while many do lose two-thirds or 66% of their excess weight, overall, we are not able to achieve that target for all patients. On average, our patients are losing between 50% and 60% of their excess weight. This is the reality. Still, it doesn't hurt to have a target that is a little ahead of your normal reach. That way we keep working with you to get to that target.

If you do succeed in losing two-thirds of your excess weight, the next target we have set on LapBase is to have you reach a BMI of 27. We have selected this target because, although you are still in the overweight category (BMI 25–30), anyone with a BMI below 27 is generally seen to be free of the risks of the diseases of obesity and the risk of premature death. An exception to this is those who have type 2 diabetes, who are better off with as low a weight as they can achieve. For the rest, a BMI of 27 puts you into a medically safe area.

The final target we set on LapBase is for you to reach a BMI of 25. You are now of normal weight. You have lost 100% of your excess weight. This is a very fine achievement, of which you should be proud. However, for most people, there is no clear health benefit in that final burst of weight loss. It tends to be of cosmetic benefit rather than a medical benefit—you look great but you may not be any healthier. Very few will reach this target and it is age-related. Our teenagers can do it but if you are over 40 it is very unlikely. Nevertheless, if you can achieve it, we are delighted for you. If you happen to be a diabetic, it is also a very real health benefit for you.

All of these targets are automatically available for you on LapBase and we are keen to share the targets with you. If you do not know where you are going, you are not going to know if and when you get there. However, we must be realistic and we must acknowledge the very important benefits of even a small weight loss. On average, the weight loss will be between 50% and 60% of excess weight. Many people will lose more and many will lose less. It is well established that even a weight loss of 25% of excess weight leads to an improvement in health and quality of life. We would be disappointed if this was all we achieved, but it can happen and sometimes we are forced to accept limited benefits. As a general rule, we regard a weight loss of less than 25% of excess weight as being unsatisfactory and for these people we implement our "intensive care pathway" to get them to a better level. Losing between 25% and 50% of excess weight is acceptable and worthwhile but rather ordinary and we would be constantly looking for improvement on this loss. Any weight loss of more the 50% of excess weight is good. It provides major health advantages, a longer life and a better quality of life. We will be pushing you steadily until you have achieved at least that amount.

HOW QUICKLY WILL I LOSE IT?

We prefer a steady progression of gentle weight loss for between 18 months and 3 years.

We all seek instant gratification. We want what we want immediately, if not sooner. Not so with the LAP-BAND™. A great strength of the LAP-BAND™ compared to early forms of weight loss surgery, such as stomach stapling, is that the weight loss occurs in a sensible way. We have control. The band is adjustable. We set the effect on satiety through adjusting the band. We tailor that setting to achieve a steady progression of weight loss, not a sudden drop.

With weight loss surgery in the past, such as gastric bypass and other forms of stomach stapling, we had no control of the settings after we had finished the operation and left the operating room. What was set during the stapling procedure had to be correct forever. It had to be loose enough that the person could eat and drink in the days immediately after the procedure and yet still act as an effective restriction on eating 10 years later. This is just not possible. The body changes, it adapts and what was initially quite tight becomes looser. In order to seek some long-term control on weight, the settings were often made very tight at the start, leading to a very rapid weight loss during the first 6 months. There was a loss of considerable amount of muscle as well as a loss of fat. This is not at all what we want. There was some further weight loss for up to 12 months but generally that was all. Whatever you had lost at 12 months was about all that you were going to lose. As a result, it was often a tough first 12 months, with good weight loss but not a good quality of life, with very little food intake and plenty of vomiting. The weight then tended to remain stable for 2 or 3 more years. After that there was a slow progression of weight gain and there was not much we or you could do to stop it.

We do not seek this pattern of rapid weight loss with the LAP-BAND™. There is good evidence that rapid weight loss is unhealthy. We are seeking changes for a lifetime and we prefer to attain these changes steadily over at least 18 months. For some people, there is a more rapid weight loss and, as long as there are no problems, such as vomiting or severe limitations on eating, we do not interfere. But we are not going to push you to achieve that by further adjusting while the weight loss is progressing. The adjustment is determined largely by the weight loss. If you are progressing well with good weight loss, with no negative symptoms and you are not feeling hungry or eating too much at mealtimes, we see you as being in the green zone (see Chapter 8) and allow you to progress. If, however, the weight loss is slow, you are getting hungry and eating too easily, we see you as being in the yellow zone and in need of further adjustments.

The average BMI of all of our patients is approximately 45. If you are at about this level, we would expect you to lose half of your excess weight by the end of the first year and to lose two-thirds of your excess weight by 18 months. This will easily be achieved if, on average, you lose about 2.2 lb (1 kg) per week in the first 6 months after placement of the band and then an average of 1.1 lb (0.5 kg) per week over the next year.

However, these expectations are very dependent on your initial BMI. If you have a very high BMI, such as 70 or 80, you have many more pounds (kilograms) to lose and this will take longer, but the number of pounds (kilograms) lost per weeks will be higher. We would be expecting a weight loss of 4.4 lb (2 kg) or more per week initially and we would expect that it will take 3 years or even more to get to the target of losing two-thirds of excess weight. If you are relatively slim, maybe a BMI of 34, you will lose fewer pounds (kilograms) per week but should achieve that target of two-thirds of excess weight lost by 12 months or even less.

This is where the LapBase software helps us a great deal. On the screen we can see if you are on track to these targets or if you are moving too slowly. Weight loss is never constant. In some weeks it seems easy and in other weeks, even though you believe that you are following all the rules, you just don't seem to move. That happens. With LapBase, we can tell if, overall, you are on track to the targets. If you are, we can reassure you even if it has been a slow week. If you are not, we can look for a reason and hopefully we can correct whatever is not optimal.

COULD I FAIL TO LOSE ENOUGH WEIGHT?

Of course. Nothing is perfect and, while the vast majority of the people we treat will experience a good weight loss, there are some for whom we have not achieved enough. You are not happy and we are not happy. We will always be keen to work hard with you to resolve the problem. Over the years and with experience of looking after thousands of patients, we have learnt much about why some people get better results than others. We certainly don't know everything yet and we cannot be sure we can succeed with every-body but, for most of those who are not doing well, we can identify possible causes and usually we can correct them.

If we can see that you are not progressing as well as we had hoped, we move you to our "intensive care" program. This includes an analysis of all the possible causes for a poor outcome, correction of those that we can correct and an increased frequency of visits to optimize the adjustments. We also would increase the support for good eating practices and push for more exercise and increases in the activities of daily living.

WHAT MUST I DO TO GET THE BEST WEIGHT LOSS?

The best results after placement of the LAP-BAND™ will occur when there is a partnership between you and your surgeon.

The surgeon has a range of responsibilities and tasks that must be done properly and you have a range of responsibilities and tasks that you must do properly.

If we both fulfill our part of the partnership, we can almost always achieve reasonable outcomes.

These roles in the partnership have been listed in Chapter 4 but we will repeat them here for your benefit.

SURGEON'S THREE COMMITMENTS

1. To place the band correctly and safely.
2. To ensure the patient is able to access good follow-up.
3. To teach the patient the rules to follow to fulfill their role.

PATIENT'S THREE COMMITMENTS

1. To follow the rules regarding eating and drinking, as discussed in Chapter 6.

2. To follow the rules regarding exercise and activity, as discussed in Chapter 7.

3. To come back for follow-up permanently with visits at least once every 6 months.

If we both fulfill our tasks optimally you will be able to achieve good weight loss, better health, and an improved quality and length of life. It is certainly worth the effort.

PATIENT ANECDOTE REBECCA BOUTSIKOUDIS

 I have tried all the diets from A to Z. I was usually able to lose some, but always gained it back the minute I went off of the plan. I have always had problems with portion control. I might eat the right things, but in mega-size portions. I was a big carb eater too, so when I did the low-carb diet, it was such a drastic change that I could not stick to it.

The plans were too hard for me to stick with on any long-term basis. I became more and more isolated, uncomfortable and embarrassed about my appearance as the weight just packed on. Physically, I panted going up a flight of stairs, had no energy, was taking full-blown asthma medicine, had knee and back pain, and severe chronic heartburn. I felt like my body was falling apart and my life along with it. Although I am considered a "people person" by many, my self-esteem was very low. I was miserable. When my eating and weight were out of control, I felt like my whole life was out of control.

My father, a physician, told me about the LAP-BAND™ and encouraged me to look into it. He has seen me struggle all my life with my weight. I knew about the gastric bypass, but ruled that out as too invasive, with too many complications and the possibility of too many nutritional issues. I read about people who had to take vitamin B_{12} shots for the rest of their lives. I wanted something as close to natural as I could get.

I began researching the LAP-BAND™ and joined several groups so I could read about everyone's experiences—positive and negative. I basically learned that if you are ready and willing to commit to a new lifestyle, the LAP-BAND™ is for you. I was definitely ready. I liked the fact that the procedure carried minimal risk and was reversible. I also liked the fact that it was adjustable to each person's needs. This is not a "cookie cutter" operation. The principle of the LAP-BAND™ is so simple, yet so effective. Restrict the amount you can eat, but still feel full while only eating a little. The less you eat, the less calories consumed, and *voila* … painless weight loss.

I made the commitment and had the operation. I was scared at first that I would not succeed, but I had the right positive mental attitude. I followed the advice of my nutritionist and physicians very closely. After the weight started coming off at a steady pace I started feeling confident that I could do this and *the band really does work, I am doing this and I am not hungry!!!* I knew I was in control of my eating finally, at last. It has given me the confidence to know I will not gain the weight back as I did every time before.

I lost 110 pounds (50 kg) and I have gone from a tight size 26 to a size 6 petite. I have never looked back, only forward enjoying my new life. Physically, my back and knee pain have disappeared, my heartburn has disappeared and I am only taking one asthma medication. I can walk 2 miles (3.2 km) without thinking about it and even enjoy it now. Emotionally, I have more self-confidence and have the energy to concentrate on having a life that is not centered around food. I can center it around my family, career and friends.

I have the need to share the LAP-BAND™ with anyone I come across that is struggling with weight loss. I want to tell everyone that this is the one thing that works and keeps working. It does not go away; it does not allow you to "fall off the wagon."

It is a consistent reminder that I made a decision to control my eating and live a healthy lifestyle.

I feel a sense of freedom in my new body. I live comfortably and with the confidence knowing each day I am in control.

Would I have the surgery for the LAP-BAND™ again? In a heartbeat. I wish I had taken control earlier in life. Now that I have, the world is at my doorstep!!

THE GOLDEN RULES OF EATING AND EXERCISE

The eight golden rules

1. Eat three or less small meals per day.
2. Do not eat anything between meals.
3. Eat slowly and stop when no longer hungry.
4. Focus on nutritious foods.
5. Avoid calorie-containing liquids.
6. Exercise for at least 30 minutes every day.
7. Be active throughout each day.
8. Always keep in contact with us.

THE EIGHT GOLDEN RULES

We have formulated eight "golden rules" for getting the best result from the procedure. It is of vital importance that you follow these rules. The success of the procedure requires us to place the band correctly, but it equally requires that you follow these rules.

We have been tempted to call them guidelines rather than rules. They are not absolute. A thunderbolt will not come from the heavens and strike you down if you break one of them. And, almost certainly, every patient has at one time or another broken each of the rules.

However, they are more than guidelines. They do need to be followed to get the best results. If you do transgress one of them, we want you to feel guilty, admit to your sins and work out how you will avoid doing something so terrible ever again.

But do remember that if the band is not correctly adjusted you will not be able to follow the rules. You must be in the green zone (see Chapter 8) to follow them. So, before being consumed by self-loathing at your weakness, do consider if correcting the adjustment of the band is needed and come in to talk to us about it.

We have already discussed these rules in the preceding chapters. In this chapter these rules are restated as a condensation of the advice in the earlier chapters. We are repeating the key elements of the advice. We state the rules and briefly expand on what each rule intends. If you are unsure about what they mean, reread Chapters 6–8 on eating, exercise and adjustment and, if still unclear, talk to us.

THE EIGHT GOLDEN RULES

1. Eat three or less small meals per day.

2. Do not eat anything between meals.

3. Eat slowly and stop when no longer hungry.

4. Focus on nutritious foods.

5. Avoid calorie-containing liquids.

6. Exercise for at least 30 minutes every day.

7. Be active throughout the day.

8. Always keep in contact with us.

---

1. EAT THREE OR LESS SMALL MEALS PER DAY

The LAP-BAND™ works primarily by taking away your appetite. If it is adjusted correctly you should not feel hungry. You may eat up to three times a day. We don't mind if you eat less than three times per day. Many people do not feel like breakfast and some will miss a midday meal. If you don't feel inclined to eat, don't eat. If you find you are getting hungry between meals, tell us. We will probably consider adjusting the band a little tighter.

There is not much room for food as there is a virtual stomach rather than a real space above the band. As you eat, the food seeks a space and you need to keep that space quite small. Therefore, each meal should be about the amount of food you can get into half a glass. If you eat more than that you will not lose weight so easily and you will gradually stretch the stomach. This can lead to the need for further surgery later on to reduce the enlarged stomach.

The adjustability of the band is the key to allowing you to be happy with this small amount of food. If you find that you are tending to eat more than that, tell us and we will consider adding more fluid to the band. Always use a small plate, put a small amount of food on the plate, and always try to leave some. Remember the angels. They need their share.

2. DO NOT EAT ANYTHING BETWEEN MEALS

No snacks, no biscuits with your coffee, no fruit, nothing. All food must be restricted to mealtimes. One of the most frequent causes for failure is snacking between meals. If you are getting hungry between meals and are tempted to have a snack, you must tell us. It is probably due to inadequate adjustment and you may need more fluid added to the band. Between meals you can only have zero-calorie liquids—water, mineral water, tea, coffee or low-calorie soft drinks.

3. EAT SLOWLY AND STOP WHEN NO LONGER HUNGRY

When you have eaten enough you will no longer be hungry and signals from your stomach to your brain tell you that you do not need any more. These signals take time to be generated. Give them that time. Each meal should be stretched out over 15–20 minutes. If you eat rapidly you will already have eaten too much before you realize that you have had enough. However, do not eat beyond 30 minutes. Throw away whatever you haven't eaten at that time. That is the end of that meal and you must have nothing else until the next meal.

Try to make each meal last for 15–20 minutes. Try to sense when you have had enough and stop before you feel at all uncomfortable. Use a small plate, put a small amount of food on the plate, and develop the habit of always leaving some of it uneaten.

Once the meal is finished it is essential that you take no further food until the next mealtime. This has to be avoided absolutely. The slow emptying of the stomach gives you a feeling of fullness, which should make it easy for you to achieve this. You must ensure that this indeed does happen.

4. FOCUS ON NUTRITIOUS FOODS

Foods that are high in protein (e.g. meats, especially fish, eggs, dairy products, lentils, beans, nuts) and foods that are high in complex carbohydrates (e.g. vegetables, some cereals) are best. Simple sugars are worst. Be careful with foods that are high in fats as they are a dense form of calories. Be careful with fruits as they contain quite a lot of sugar.

The good foods can come from all the main food groups and include vegetables, meats, eggs, cereals and dairy. There is no need to focus unduly on the particular foods in fine detail. It is not rocket science. It is simply selecting foods that are good (protein and complex carbohydrates), being careful with those that are not so good (fats, alcohol) and avoiding those that are bad (simple sugars). And take a well-balanced vitamin and mineral replacement each day.

5. AVOID CALORIE-CONTAINING LIQUIDS

Any calorie-containing liquids will tend to flow past the restriction of the band and not give you any feeling of satiety. You are then more likely to take too much. You are only allowed to drink:

- water
- mineral water
- tea or coffee (with low-fat milk if you wish but no sugar)
- low-calorie soft drinks (but be careful with the gas).

The exceptions to the "no liquid calorie" rule are a glass of wine with meals, which we know is good for your health and good for your weight loss when taken in a modest amount, and up to 1 pint (500 mL) of low-fat milk each day.

6. EXERCISE FOR AT LEAST 30 MINUTES EACH DAY

This is at least as important as all of the other rules. Not only must you take in less calories but you must also use up more calories. Exercise will improve your general health as well. Initially, while you are severely obese this can be difficult, but, as your weight decreases, it becomes easier. As you become fitter and healthier, you get greater enjoyment from exercise.

We understand that not everybody is sports minded and exercise may be something quite new for you. Start slowly and seek to build up activity progressively. Aim to put together 30 minutes or more of moderate-intensity physical activity on most and preferably all days. Walking is ideal to start off with. As your fitness improves, progress to more vigorous walking and even jogging, cycling, aerobics, swimming, and light resistance training. As your weight comes down your exercise capacity will increase and your general activities during the day will increase. This is to be encouraged, and the more active you are the better the result will be.

Your exercise program should be aerobic. You should be puffing and, if you check your pulse, generally it should be up around 120–140 beats per minute. There are a wide range of activities that will allow you to achieve this. If you can manage it, a personal trainer or fitness consultant can be an excellent assistant. They can provide an individual program according to your specific preferences and lifestyle that is realistic and achievable. Regular exercise requires commitment. The more effort you put in, the greater benefits you will see and feel.

7. BE ACTIVE THROUGHOUT EACH DAY

Think of movement and activity as opportunities and not as an inconvenience. Try to be active every day in as many ways as you can. Make it a habit to walk or cycle instead of using the car. Become active in the garden and do things yourself instead of using machines. Avoid sitting down at all cost. You should see sitting down as an opportunity for activity lost.

Try to spend as much time outdoors as possible. We tend to be more active when outdoors. Use a pedometer as a stimulus to show you how your activity level is increasing. If you are using a pedometer, aim to get beyond 10,000 steps per day—this represents a very good level of routine daily activity.

8. ALWAYS KEEP IN CONTACT WITH US

We want to follow you permanently. There will never be a time when we say that the job of controlling your obesity is done and we do not need to see you anymore. There will always be a need to check your progress, monitor your health, check for nutritional deficiencies, make sure that you understand the rules, bring you up to date with new developments, and adjust the volume of fluid in the band.

There is always going to be a very small loss of fluid from the band over time. For example, if you had 3 mL of fluid present and we checked the volume after a 6-month period, there would probably be about 2.7 mL present. This occurs because the balloon of the band is not totally impermeable. If 3 mL was the correct volume, you would be starting to get hungry and eat more with a volume of 2.7 mL. It is important you understand that this can happen and come back to see us for replacement of that small fluid loss. This is the main reason that we want a maximum of 6 months between appointments.

FREQUENTLY ASKED QUESTIONS

CHAPTER ELEVEN

SHOULD I EXPECT A LOT OF VOMITING?

There really should be no vomiting at all. The procedure is designed to place a gentle restriction on your eating. If you find that you are vomiting, then either there is something wrong with the settings of the band or there is something wrong with your following of the rules regarding eating. It is important not to have frequent vomiting as this could lead to shifting of the stomach within the band and compromise the outcome. Ideally there would be no vomiting at all.

WHAT SHOULD I DO IF I DO GET VOMITING FOR OTHER REASONS?

Of course, you are at risk of having vomiting, just as anyone else might, from food poisoning, gastroenteritis, pregnancy or for numerous other reasons. Curiously, it has not proved to be at all common and rarely has it been a problem. Your first task is prevention. Avoid eating or drinking potentially contaminated food or water. This is particularly important when you are traveling. If you start vomiting and feel it may continue, seek medical help to stop it as quickly as possible. If it continues, contact the clinic and have some fluid removed from the band. Once you start vomiting a lot, there is swelling of the stomach inside the band, making it tighter. The swelling perpetuates the vomiting. Removing fluid breaks that cycle.

WILL I BE CONSTIPATED?

You may be. It is inevitable that, as you eat less food, then you eat less fiber, and your bowel activity will decrease. However, we have been pleasantly surprised to find that this has not proved to be a common problem at all. If you do become constipated, it is acceptable to take one of the bulk-forming laxatives, such as Metamucil, with plenty of water and this should correct the problem.

SHOULD I TAKE A VITAMIN SUPPLEMENT?

Yes. You may well be getting sufficient vitamins from the food that you are able to take, but as you lose weight you have a particular need for additional vitamins and, therefore, we strongly recommend that you do take a multivitamin supplement. It is particularly important that the supplement has sufficient folate and iron. We will monitor specific vitamins and minerals, such as vitamin B_{12} and folate and iron, each year after operation to see if any deficiency in these is occurring. If there is, specific addition of these will be recommended.

WHAT ABOUT OTHER TABLETS AND MEDICINES?

In general you will continue to take the medications prescribed. However, if they are in the form of a bulky tablet, it may be necessary to break them up. Try them out. If they feel as if they tend to stick at the bottom of the esophagus, you may have to crush them up and take them with some yogurt to disguise the taste. However, if you are going to do this, check with your pharmacist first. Quite a number of tablets are specially formulated to be slowly released or released further down the gut and not in the stomach. It would be important to clarify this first. Capsules should not be a problem to swallow as they are designed to soften and melt inside the body.

WHAT HAPPENS IF I BECOME PREGNANT?

We have now had many pregnancies in our patients and it has been all good news. The band itself does not interfere in any negative way with the pregnancy. The likelihood of becoming pregnant is probably higher because, having lost weight, your periods are often more regular. The adjustability of the band makes managing the pregnancy much easier because we can remove some fluid from the band if you have a lot of vomiting early in the pregnancy or if you are not putting on enough weight for you and the baby during the pregnancy. Normally, we will adjust the volume of fluid in the band early in the pregnancy to ensure that there is optimal nutritional intake for both yourself and the baby. Even if you put on some weight during the pregnancy, we can tighten it up again later and get that weight off again.

IS THE SILICONE DANGEROUS TO ME?

We have no information to suggest that it is. We have been using silicone implants in various areas of surgery for more than 50 years. There were concerns and a lot of legal actions raised regarding the liquid silicone used in breast implants. However, this turned out to be more of a political and legal dispute than a true medical problem as a review of a large number of high-quality medical studies were unable to show that what was being claimed was true.

The LAP-BAND™ is made of solid silicone and has no liquid component. Therefore, it cannot leak into the tissues in the way that liquid silicone possibly could. We expect the likelihood of any problem is extremely low. However, it could be that information about problems relevant to this question may become available in the future. If they do, we would let you know.

HOW LONG WILL THE BAND LAST?

We really don't know. We have been using the LAP-BAND™ for more than 10 years and there has been no sign of it wearing out. However, realistically we can't expect a device such as this to last 40–50 years. We do expect that somewhere down the track there will be failure of the adjusting balloon, in particular, and should this occur, the band would need to be replaced. It is going to remain to be determined if and when this should be necessary. We are hopeful that you will get good service from the LAP-BAND™ for at least 20 years and if, after that, we have to replace it, well so be it.

CAN THE BAND BE REMOVED?

Yes. It can be removed quite easily. It is not our intention to ever remove it, but should it become appropriate for whatever reason, then it can be removed. If it has been placed laparoscopically, then it can be removed laparoscopically. After the band has been removed, we would expect the stomach to go back to normal.

However, if the band was removed and no other effective method for weight control was instituted, we would expect that you would put back on the weight that you had lost. It might happen slowly but it is most likely that over a 2-year period you would return to your original weight.

WHAT DO I DO WHEN DINING OUT?

Because of the limited capacity of your new "virtual" stomach, you must restrict yourself generally to an appetizer (an entrée in Australia). Eat slowly while those with you are overeating with two or three courses. Social eating is one setting where we will excuse you from the 30-minute rule. Because these occasions may go on for some hours, we recommend that you pick very slowly at your food over this time. Push it around the plate and nibble at it.

If you are visiting friends, it is probably better to advise the host or hostess that you can only eat a small amount to save embarrassment when you reject most of their carefully prepared food.

WHAT ABOUT ALCOHOL?

Alcohol has a high calorie content and is a liquid and therefore, in theory, should be discouraged. However, there are health advantages in a modest alcohol intake, particularly of wine. And we have found from our research that modest alcohol intake is associated with improved weight loss. We therefore are happy to let you have up to seven standard drinks a week, or an average of one drink per day. Note that this is not a requirement; it is the upper limit.

WILL I NEED PLASTIC SURGERY FOR EXCESS SKIN FOLDS ONCE I HAVE LOST WEIGHT?

Generally no. About a quarter of our patients need to have something done. The most common need is for the removal of the abdominal apron. Generally, we don't want you to consider any plastic surgery until about 2 years after the procedure. Usually there is enough elasticity in the skin to take up the slack sufficiently and we would like to wait to see how effective this is before considering plastic surgery.

WHAT SHOULD HAPPEN IF I DEVELOP ANOTHER ILLNESS?

A real advantage with the LAP-BAND™ is its adjustability. If you have some other illness that makes it inappropriate to have restriction on food intake, then the fluid can easily be removed and there would be very little limitation on nutrition. Once you have recovered from the illness, even if you have put on weight, the fluid can be added and the original status can be restored.

CAN I BURP WITH THE LAP-BAND™?

Not so easily. As we eat we always swallow air and normally we would bring this back up again quite unconsciously. The band interferes with this easy bringing up of wind. It is common in the first few weeks after the procedure for people to notice a difficulty with bloating and the feeling that they want to burp but cannot. This rarely seems to persist as a problem months later. We presume that the stomach below the band changes its shape enough to reduce the problem but for whatever reason it does not seem to continue to be troublesome.

HOW ARE THE ADJUSTMENTS TO THE BAND DONE?

We generally will start tightening the band at 4 weeks after the initial operation. The adjustment is almost always performed in the office at the time of consultation. It does not require any anesthetic. It consists of passing a fine needle through the skin into the access port. It only takes a few minutes to do and is not usually associated with significant discomfort. On occasions it will need to be performed in the radiology department where we can see more accurately where the access port is.

We will generally adjust the band every 2 weeks until we feel that we have the right setting. This may take four or five adjustments. Once the correct setting is reached we would leave it at that level as long as the rate of weight loss initially, and then the weight maintenance later on, was satisfactory. Additional adjustments can occur whenever necessary. When you reach the goal weight, we leave the setting at that level so as to maintain that weight. If we reduced the setting at this time you would expect to find an increase in your weight.

ARE THE ADJUSTMENTS VERY PAINFUL?

No, they are not. Some people worry more about the adjustments before they are done than they worried about the operation. This is really quite inappropriate. Each adjustment consists of a jab with a needle and then some mild discomfort as we push on the access port. It usually only takes 2 or 3 minutes and doesn't require any local anesthetic. It would hurt as much to have the local anesthetic put in as it does to have the whole adjustment. After you have your first adjustment you will be reassured and no longer need to worry.

IS THIS COSMETIC SURGERY?

No. It is not. Obesity is a potentially severe and, in fact, a life-threatening disease and this procedure is for treatment of this disease. The disease is present when the BMI is greater than 30. It is recognized as such by your health funds and by governmental agencies involved in health. While there are undoubted benefits to your appearance with weight loss, the primary reason for us doing the procedure is for the health benefit.

WHAT HAPPENS IF I GO OVERSEAS OR TO REMOTE LOCATIONS?

Generally there is no problem. You really don't want to get into any difficulties while away and therefore you have to be doubly careful to follow the rules regarding the type of food you eat. Take this book with you and, should you need any medical care while traveling, this will give the physicians where you are much of the information that they would need to understand what has been done. We would hope that they would telephone us and discuss the problem before they interfered in any way with the device.

IS AIRPLANE TRAVEL A PROBLEM?

It can be more difficult to eat when flying. There are often little bubbles of air in the balloon of the LAP-BAND™. We try to flush these out when we initially prime the band but we cannot clear them all. Generally they don't matter. However, when you are at 35,000 feet in a plane that is only partially pressurized, these bubbles may expand enough to make the band tighter. You may find that you have difficulty with solid foods and even with liquids. If so, just relax and enjoy the trip. Watch the movie instead of having lunch. When you return to ground level, the bubbles will shrink down and you will be back to normal.

REFERENCES

1. Yach D, Stuckler D, Brownell K. Epidemiologic and economic consequences of the global epidemics of obesity and diabetes. *Nat Med* 2006; 12(1):62–66.
2. Mokdad AH, Marks JS, Stroup DF, Gerberding JL. Actual causes of death in the United States, 2000. *JAMA* 2004; 291(10):1238–1245.
3. Flegal KM, Graubard BI, Williamson DF, Gail MH. Excess deaths associated with underweight, overweight, and obesity. *JAMA* 2005; 293(15):1861–1867.
4. Colditz GA, Willett WC, Rotnitzky A, Manson JE. Weight gain as a risk factor for clinical diabetes mellitus in women. *Ann Intern Med* 1995; 122(7):481–486.
5. Dixon JB, O'Brien P. Health outcomes of severely obese type 2 diabetic subjects 1 year after laparoscopic adjustable gastric banding. *Diabetes Care* 2002; 25(2):358–363.
6. O'Brien PE, Brown WA, Dixon JB. Obesity, weight loss and bariatric surgery. *Med J Aust* 2005; 183(6):310–314.
7. Dixon JB, O'Brien PE. Lipid profile in the severely obese: changes with weight loss after lap-band surgery. *Obes Res* 2002; 10(9):903–910.
8. Dixon JB, O'Brien PE. Gastroesophageal reflux in obesity: the effect of lap-band placement. *Obes Surg* 1999; 9(6):527–531.
9. Dixon JB, Schachter LM, O'Brien PE. Sleep disturbance and obesity: changes following surgically induced weight loss. *Arch Intern Med* 2001; 161(1):102–106.
10. Dixon JB, Schachter LM, O'Brien PE. Polysomnography before and after weight loss in obese patients with severe sleep apnea. *Int J Obes Relat Metab Disord* 2005; 29(9):1048–1054.
11. Dixon JB, Chapman L, O'Brien P. Marked improvement in asthma after Lap-Band surgery for morbid obesity. *Obes Surg* 1999; 9(4):385–389.

12. Dixon JB, Bhathal PS, Hughes NR, O'Brien PE. Nonalcoholic fatty liver disease: improvement in liver histological analysis with weight loss. *Hepatology* 2004; 39(6):1647–1654.

13. Dixon JB, O'Brien PE. Neck circumference a good predictor of raised insulin and free androgen index in obese premenopausal women: changes with weight loss. *Clin Endocrinol (Oxf)* 2002; 57(6):769–778.

14. Dixon JB, Dixon ME, O'Brien PE. Birth outcomes in obese women after laparoscopic adjustable gastric banding. *Obstet Gynecol* 2005; 106(5):965–972.

15. Dixon JB, Dixon ME, O'Brien PE. Depression in association with severe obesity: changes with weight loss. *Arch Intern Med* 2003; 163(17):2058–2065.

16. Dixon JB, Dixon ME, O'Brien PE. Quality of life after lap-band placement: influence of time, weight loss, and comorbidities. *Obes Res* 2001; 9(11):713–721.

17. Glenny AM, O'Meara S, Melville A, Sheldon TA, Wilson C. The treatment and prevention of obesity: a systematic review of the literature. *Int J Obes Relat Metab Disord* 1997; 21(9):715–737.

18. Li Z, Maglione M, Tu W, et al. Meta-analysis: pharmacologic treatment of obesity. *Ann Intern Med* 2005; 142(7):532–546.

19. Van Gaal LF, Rissanen AM, Scheen AJ, Ziegler O, Rossner S. Effects of the cannabinoid-1 receptor blocker rimonabant on weight reduction and cardiovascular risk factors in overweight patients: 1-year experience from the RIO-Europe study. *Lancet* 2005; 365(9468):1389–1397.

20. O'Brien PE, McPhail T, Chaston TB, Dixon JB. Systemic review of medium term weight loss after bariatric operations. *Obes Surg* 2006; 16(8):1032–1040.

21. Chapman A, Kiroff G, Game P, et al. Laparoscopic adjustable gastric banding in the treatment of obesity: a systematic review. *Surgery* 2004; 135:326–351.

22. O'Brien PE, Dixon J, Laurie C, et al. Treatment of mild to moderate obesity with laparoscopic adjustable gastric banding or an intensive medical program: a randomized trial. *Ann Intern Med* 2006; 144:625–633.

INDEX